Learning to Care
on the
PSYCHIATRIC WARD

Martin F. Ward
RMN, DN(Lond), CertEd (Leeds), RNT, NEBSSDip

Psychiatric Nurse Tutor, Broadland School of Nursing,
Hellesdon Hospital, Norwich

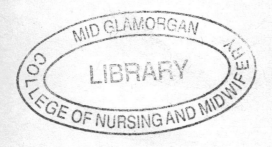
Edward Arnold
A division of Hodder & Stoughton
LONDON   MELBOURNE   AUCKLAND

© 1986 M. Ward

First published in Great Britain 1986
Reprinted 1990

British Library Cataloguing in Publication Data

Ward, Martin F.
  Learning to care on the psychiatric ward.
  – (Learning to care series)
  1. Psychiatric nursing
  I. Title
  610.73′68   RC440

Whilst the advice and information in this book is believed to be
true and accurate at the date of going to press, neither the author
nor the publisher can accept any legal responsibility or liability for
any errors or omissions that may be made.

Typeset in 10/11 pt Trump Mediaeval by Rowland Phototypesetting
Ltd. Printed and bound in Great Britain for Edward Arnold, a
division of Hodder and Stoughton Limited, Mill Road, Dunton
Green, Sevenoaks, Kent TN13 2YA by Clays Ltd, St Ives plc.

CONTENTS

Editors' foreword iv
Preface iv

1 Introduction 1

2 Peter, who seems anxious 21

3 Wendy, who is depressed 36

4 Alan, who is sometimes aggressive and violent 54

5 Diana, whose behaviour is designed to gain attention 68

6 Grace, who is obsessional 84

7 Isobel, who is highly suspicious and severely disturbed 98

8 Tony, who is highly over-active 115

9 George, who has been in hospital for many years 130

10 Constance, an elderly lady 146

11 The Community 162

Index 172

EDITORS' FOREWORD

In most professions there is a traditional gulf between theory and its practice, and nursing is no exception. The gulf is perpetuated when theory is taught in a theoretical setting and practice is taught by the practitioner.

This inherent gulf has to be bridged by students of nursing, and publication of this series is an attempt to aid such bridge building.

It aims to help relate theory and practice in a meaningful way whilst underlining the importance of the person being cared for.

It aims to introduce students of nursing to some of the more common problems found in each new area of experience in which they will be asked to work.

It aims to de-mystify some of the technical language they will hear, putting it in context, giving it meaning and enabling understanding.

PREFACE

As many as 5.5 million people in England and Wales suffer from some form of mental illness, many of the more serious cases being admitted to a psychiatric ward at some point or other. Whilst there they will receive specialist care and when recovered most will return to society to lead perfectly normal lives once again. Some will remain in hospital for longer periods of time and on discharge will need continuing care and support if they are to lead as full a life as possible.

Despite the large numbers involved, psychiatry remains something of a mystery both to the general public and many other health care professionals. What then is psychiatry? This book, designed for the nurse just beginning in the profession, looks at the way psychiatric illness affects people's behaviour and gives an insight into the special role played by nurses in aiding the individual's recovery. Its aim is to remove some of the mystery from psychiatry, and in particular from psychiatric patients. Obviously it cannot hope to portray all the various aspects of psychiatric behaviour for they are as varied as the people who suffer from them. What it can do, however, is to look at some of the more common problems and the wide range of interventions and strategies used by today's psychiatric nurse whilst examining the modern concept of including the individual as much as possible in his own care. Each chapter is a small story combining the problems faced by one particular individual with the care, using the nursing process, involved in their management.

Introduction

One of the major problems of starting to work on a psychiatric ward or returning to it after some absence is that clinically and professionally it is like no other nursing specialty. This book is designed both to consider why this is the case and to contrast various approaches that you might make towards individual psychiatric patients, so that you are better equipped to participate more confidently in their progress through their own illness.

Chapters 2–10 will look at a series of patients, their histories, behavioural presentations, expectations of hospitalisation and care. Before reading them, let us outline the answers to some of the more commonly asked questions about psychiatric nursing.

They are likely to centre around the following items, though not necessarily in the same order: personal; personnel; patients; role; environmental; administration; psychiatry.

Personal

'I am worried about the experience because I will not know what to do or how to behave. Am I likely to feel awkward and out of place?'
The simple answer is, no one expects you to have the answers, so do not try to be someone different because you are in a psychiatric setting. Your activities should be carefully controlled and there will always be someone on hand to help you should you get into difficulties.

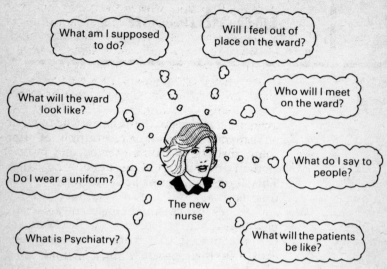

The new nurse's dilemma

What am I supposed to do?

Will I feel out of place on the ward?

What will the ward look like?

Who will I meet on the ward?

Do I wear a uniform?

What do I say to people?

The new nurse

What is Psychiatry?

What will the patients be like?

Personnel

'Who am I likely to meet? Do the same people work in a psychiatric hospital as in other hospitals?'

There are many similarities between psychiatric and general areas. The nursing structure is equivalent to that of a general hospital, both at nurse manager and ward staff level. However, it is true to say that fewer power differentials are present in psychiatry and because of the nature of the team approach used within the specialty staff are encouraged to work with the emphasis on responsibility rather than status.

There are the same medical staff though; they will be psychiatrists or trainees but all with their medical qualifications. There will be a high proportion of non-medical specialists who have a large contribution to play in the patient's daily life including in particular: clinical psychologists, occupational therapists of different types, social workers, rehabilitation staff, and community psychiatric nurses.

'How do I talk to these people?'
Talking to people who work in psychiatry is usually a far easier experience than in other clinical areas. There is a greater degree of informality and everyone is considered to have a contribution to make in the caring process.

All grades of nursing staff are expected to participate in the team approach to care which may involve anything from discussing your own observations with senior medical staff, to verbalising your own ideas within an open ward meeting of nursing/medical staff and patients. You will find these people approachable, but remember to 'be yourself'.

Patients

'What are the patients going to be like?'
Psychiatric patients are ordinary people who, sometimes through no fault of their own, have reached a point in their life where they experience feelings and emotions which are at variance with their environment. They often

Members of the psychiatric care team

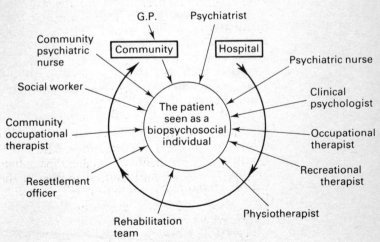

suffer extreme levels of emotion which are uncommon for the vast majority of the population. For them it can be a terrifying and lonely experience of uncertainty and confusion where life takes on a significance totally out of proportion to reality.

Sometimes it is a response to real personal problems and at other times there seems to be no obvious reason for it at all. They use the same range of behaviour patterns as everyone else, but because of the way they perceive their surroundings and life situation, appear to act in an exaggerated form of that behaviour. For instance, if you were under siege in your own home by a group of terrorists who were trying to kill you, it would be expected of you to behave in an aggressive fashion to protect yourself, your family and your belongings. No one would consider your actions out of place if you telephoned the police asking for assistance, shouted from your windows for help, barricaded yourself in and defended yourself with whatever means possible when the terrorists came to get you. In fact you would be highly commended by all concerned for your bravery, tenacity and ingenuity. In other words your aggression, your guile and your manoeuvring would all be seen as totally appropriate to the situation and completely acceptable. But what if you only imagined that terrorists were out to get you, what then of your behaviour? Would others understand why you needed to behave so aggressively? If you had the time to sit down and talk with them to explain the problem, they might understand and try to help you in some way. However, if you suspected that they too were a member of the gang, you would of course take action accordingly. In short, your behaviour, though totally acceptable to you, would not be understood by others and might be seen as unnecessary and anti-social. It would, though, be no different to that used by others in their own real life crises.

One problem facing the nurse is recognising that the behaviour itself is not normal, but the context in which it occurs is. Trying to identify its cause and then helping the patient to explore alternatives so that he can come to terms with it, is the only way to actually predict these fluctuations in behavioural response. Very rarely do patients use totally bizarre behaviour and, in fact, the vast majority behave exactly as you would if you felt as sad or as frightened as many of them do. Often, once you have established why a patient is behaving the way he is, it is quite understandable.

'Are they aggressive?'

Many psychiatric patients seem aggressive, but in fact they have lost only the ability to integrate in a socially acceptable fashion. These are usually patients of long standing. Others, of course, are very definitely aggressive and violent, often as a response to the uncertainty that they create for themselves because of their distortion of reality. In other words, what they perceive as taking place contradicts what their mind tells them should take place. At times this can seem remarkably threatening. Often it can be averted by nurses generating an unambiguous clinical environment based on equanimity, trust, warmth and understanding. It can only be achieved by trying to treat the patient as a true individual and ensuring your interactions with him are as honest and non-threatening as possible.

'Will they talk to me and will I be able to talk to them?'

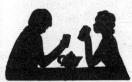

Yes, they will talk to you. Very often that is exactly what they want to do; only a very few withdraw totally and refuse to acknowledge you. There is skill in communicating effectively, however, and it only comes about through practice. One guiding rule when talking to patients is that neither of you should feel disadvantaged by the presence of the other, and if you do, then alter the interaction accordingly.

In a normal social setting, let's say a party, you would select people to talk to who were interesting, amusing, attractive, etc. You would be unlikely to talk to those who seemed eager to manipulate you into doing things you did not wish to do, who wished to extract personalised information from you, who threatened you in some way or who were simply impolite. The same rule applies in the clinical environment, though of course it is not regulated by the same motives as if you were at a party. You need to watch for the patient's response to your approach – does he seem frightened or threatened by you, shy away from you, appear worried by things you say, avoid eye contact with you or try to change the topic of conversation? If the answer is, 'yes', it could be that he sees you in the same light as the 'undesirable' at the party and someone to be steered clear of. You need to be aware of your effects upon others for it is after all your reason for being with them and caring for them. Likewise you must remember that the patient may try to take advantage of you. Just because he is a patient does not preclude him from having human emotions – far from it – and if he sees the opportunity to manipulate you into saying and doing things which are unprofessional or counter-productive, he may well decide to do so. You must, therefore, be aware of his effect upon you. If you cannot do that, using your existing communication skills, seek advice from someone in the clinical area or talk to the patient about it. You may be surprised by the answer he gives you.

'How do they get into hospital and what if they want to leave?'

Most psychiatric patients are voluntary or informal, that is they become in-patients through the normal system of medical referral and agree to admission. No one can be admitted without having been seen by a psychiatrist. A small proportion, between 10 and 15 per cent, are formal or involuntary admissions who, usually because of the severity and depersonalising nature of their condition and behaviour, are unable to make clear cut decisions concerning their health and personal safety. They are admitted under sections of the 1983 Mental Health Act and the duration, nature and purpose of each section is legally controlled. Their freedom as a consequence is restricted, and they might even be treated against their wishes if the condition warrants.

Depersonalising is the sensation of being changed as a person in some way either mentally or physically

Most patients are free to leave a psychiatric hospital in the same way as they would any other hospital, and many go home at weekends. This is not so with a detained patient who must remain until such time as his section expires (when the section may be renewed) or more likely until he is capable of making an accurate decision about himself and his life situation.

'Why are people admitted to psychiatric care?'

As already stated, only a small proportion of people who develop some form of psychiatric behaviour are actually admitted to hospital. For many it is a question of receiving support and medication from their general practitioner while carrying on their everyday lives. Others who remain in the community are referred by their general practitioner to see a psychiatrist in an out-patient clinic and may well receive more specific care either from that psychiatrist or from a community psychiatric nurse. Still others, of course, never come into contact

Psychiatric behaviour is actions, thoughts and feelings of an inappropriate or exaggerated nature experienced by some individuals in response to otherwise uncontrollable levels of stress and anxiety

with health care professionals and eventually learn to cope with the problems on their own or adapt to their difficulties with the help of relatives and friends.

Why then are a small number of people admitted? The answer must centre around several factors:

1 Whether or not the psychiatrist feels that the individual will actually benefit in terms of recovery by being admitted to hospital. Often removing the cause of the problem reduces the stress on the individual sufficiently to allow him to be able to examine what he is doing more objectively. Hopefully he will become better at making decisions about his actions which will enable him to cope more effectively when he has been discharged.

2 The degree of disturbance experienced by the individual and the severity of its effects on his ability to function as an independent person. If a person is severely disturbed, his problem may well interfere with every aspect of his daily life so that he is totally dependent on others. The pressure that this places on relatives and friends may be a necessary consideration for the psychiatrist, as will the amount of psychological suffering experienced by the individual. For instance, two people may be hearing voices (auditory hallucinations). One of them is a lonely man, something of a social outcast, who never mixes with others and leads a very limited life style. His only consolation is the voices that he hears; they keep him company and serve as someone to talk to. In the other case the voices tell him that he is evil, and say alarming and obscene things to him. He is frightened and distressed by what he hears. The first individual is not a candi-

date for admission, but the second one is.

3 Is the individual a threat to himself or others? If a person is contemplating suicide, or other forms of self harm, it would be advisable to admit him to care so that injury can be averted. Acting in an aggressive or violent manner towards others may also be considered as a reason to admit someone, but not all people who pose a threat to others are deemed to be suffering from a psychiatric problem. The final consideration must rest on whether or not an individual is capable of controlling his own actions or can appreciate the consequences of his behaviour. The old lady living alone in a terraced house who continually leaves the gas on unlit because her memory has deteriorated may not comprehend that she might cause an explosion, killing herself and others. She might need hospitalisation. A young man who threatens the same old lady in the street and steals her handbag, though equally dangerous, would not necessarily be admitted to hospital.

4 Are others likely to take advantage of the individual because he is experiencing some form of psychiatric disturbance? Very often the nature of an individual's disturbance leaves him unable to see problems and situations as they really are. This vulnerability can often have miserable consequences for him. The man who is continuously taken advantage of by his colleagues at work, but who always does their bidding because he has no wish to offend, will soon become socially withdrawn and rejected. It is possible he could become very distressed by the whole situation but be totally incapable of doing anything about it. He may well benefit from admission to hospital.

The ultimate decision as to whether or not to admit an individual remains with the psychiatrist. Sometimes that decision will be influenced, not only by the individual's behaviour, but also by the amount of support available within the community. The help and loving care of friends and relatives may well reduce the necessity to admit even the most serious of cases.

Role

'What am I supposed to do on the psychiatric ward?'
Actually this will depend largely on the approaches and philosophy of your own clinical area, but there are common practical factors. You will be expected to try to get to know your patients as real individuals through careful observations and personal contact; by taking part in the production of care and its evaluation; by becoming involved in as much clinical activity as is deemed suitable; by helping the patient to contribute towards all the elements of his care and its reduction or cessation. Above all else, you must make personal contact with your patients. Basically this entails involving yourself in their daily activities; talking with them at every possible opportunity about matters which they deem significant or relevant to their problems or care situation; accompanying them in recreational or therapeutic situations or simply acknowledging them whenever the opportunity arises. It is only through attempting to use your own personality as a therapeutic agent that relief from emotional stress and belief in themselves can be achieved. Probably one of the greatest differences between psychiatric and general nursing roles involves the method by which patient progress is achieved. It is

Therapeutic agent means using one's own personal behaviour to bring about a change for the best in the behaviour of another

important that you try to promote patient independence of you and not dependence upon you. It is a teaching role which necessitates encouraging the patients to do as much for themselves as they are capable of doing, albeit perhaps in planned and mutually agreed stages. It takes longer than if you do it for them, but the end result is a patient who has achieved personal competency through his own endeavours, with all the dignity that that entails.

'What skills will I learn?'
Throughout our lives we come into contact with many people. With some we develop friendships, with others we never seek their company again and with many we establish casual acquaintances that provide us with social contact when and if we need it. We probably never stop to ask ourselves why we respond towards others in the way that we do, nor do we consider why our feelings vary so much about those with whom we associate.

Nurses, however, are not allowed the luxury of personal choice in the question of deciding who they will care for nor are they able to dictate the frequency with which they come into contact with those for whom they care. This may cause something of a dilemma. We tend not to mix with people we find unattractive or who threaten us in some way, either physically or psychologically. We avoid those we feel we cannot trust, those who are unpredictable and those who would take advantage of us. It is the presence of such behavioural qualities, however, that has often led to an individual being admitted to a psychiatric ward and now the nurse is expected to work with him, help and teach him. Of course not all psychiatric patients are unpopular, alarming or dangerous, as much of what they say and do becomes quite understandable once its cause has been established. It is also an assumption that the individual concerned will wish to speak to the nurse simply because of what she is. There has to be some quality that the nurse can develop that will help her firstly to overcome her own natural apprehensions and secondly enable her to make contact with her patients comfortably and effectively. This quality, or group of skills, are those which she brings to nursing in her own personality. They could be described as those which enable her to form a professional relationship, and will include:

1 Showing that she cares, by sitting patiently, listening carefully to what is said, repeating phrases and words that are important, seeking clarification about issues the patient finds important.

2 Showing that she can be trusted by doing exactly what she says she will, never making promises she cannot keep and never placing the patient at a disadvantage by making him feel small or silly.

3 Showing that she accepts the patient for what he is no matter how badly he feels about himself, by not making judgements about the things he says, not criticising him or belittling him.

4 Showing that she understands the way a patient feels even though she cannot feel the same way herself, by talking about the signs or effects of his anguish, i.e. 'you obviously feel very angry about this'.

5 Showing that she expects nothing in return for her care, by spending time with patients, even though nothing is said, and not becoming irritated because of lack of progress or recovery.

6 Showing that she sees her patients as equals, by not talking down to them, or excluding them from decisions about their

own care – and communicating with them in a way that they can understand, but without patronising them, i.e. speaking *with* them, not *at* them.

This group of skills could easily be regarded as representing those which contributed to the beginning of the counselling process. Allowing a person to vent their feelings and relieve emotional tension is an essential component in the initial stages of their recovery. If the nurse is to employ these skills usefully, therefore, she must be aware of her effects upon other people and continually monitor her own behaviour, modifying it where necessary, always learning from her successes and failures. Every skill will be enhanced by bringing to bear three other elements in her personality which are almost essential – sensitivity, humour and life experience, no matter how limited.

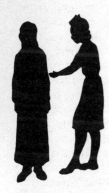

Those skills will help the nurse to establish a rapport or relationship with her patients. Once this rapport has been forged, the nurse will need other skills that she will have been taught which can be described as those enabling her to actually do something to resolve a patient's pain or suffering. The application of these skills we call nursing intervention, the method by which the nurse interrupts a chain of events to influence a change in behaviour on the part of the patient. The interruption may be small, or large, involved or simple, and may take nothing more than a nod or a smile, but it is essentially the skill of being a psychiatric nurse.

When the nurse first begins she will be expected only to develop her own skills. As she becomes more confident and adept, she will be given advice and tuition about such things as how to support and guide a patient, teach them to: make decisions about themselves without giving advice; explore problem tackling alternatives; develop their own personal effectiveness; examine their own behaviour; to relax and enjoy their lives. All this takes time and cannot be rushed for just as the patient must understand how to manage his own problems, so the nurse must understand how she managed the patient.

'What do I get out of it for myself?'
Try to get to know the patients as they really are in order to increase your confidence and ability to help them in all clinical situations. Use that experience to enhance your own personal skills, so that you are more able to generate an obviously caring and professional image for all your future patients.

Environmental

'What kind of a ward will it be? Will there be bars on the windows or padded cells?'
Old ideas about psychiatry still linger and it is difficult to convince people otherwise. Even when you tell people that such forms of restraint including strait-jackets, etc. are no longer used and, in fact, are illegal, they still seem to think that there must be at least one place in the hospital that has them. You will not find them in today's psychiatric hospitals.

The building itself can be anything from a modern unit attached to a general hospital, to one of the larger and much older traditional psychiatric hospitals. In most cases, you will find the wards are like most self-contained units with more emphasis on day facilities than sleeping ones. Day areas, therapy areas, recreational rooms and small rooms where patients can get a little peace and quiet take precedence over bedrooms or small cubicalised dormitories. Everything is done to make the rooms as comfortable and pleasing to the eye as possible. Very few patients spend waking hours in bed, and may well spend quite a long time in the ward. Thus it is important that they are made to feel relaxed but still have room to move around.

Administration

'Are psychiatric wards very strict? Do I wear a uniform?'
As already mentioned, the usual atmosphere within a psychiatric ward is relaxed and informal. The special environment needed to create positive attitudes towards personal growth and recovery would be destroyed if the patients felt they were merely observers of ward routine. The psychiatric nurse must be approachable or she is not a good psychiatric nurse. Whether you wear a uniform or not depends entirely on your hospital's philosophy, although most these days tend to be less inclined to use them. Certainly the carrying of scissors, etc. is not really justified.

Psychiatry

'What is psychiatry?'
Psychiatry is classified as that medical specialty responsible for the treatment of abnormal behaviour.

'What is mental illness?'
In our society abnormal behaviour is termed mental illness, though it is unlike any illness you will see in a general hospital as it has no obvious body changes. It can only be detected by observing the individual's overt behaviour in response to his environment, and penetrating his covert world in conversation and iden-

The covert world is a patient's hidden behaviour, i.e. his thoughts, attitudes, fears and desires

tifying his thoughts, ideas and related cognitive activities. A simplistic description of mental illness would be 'an extraordinary response to an ordinary stimulus'.

As we grow, our personalities grow with us. The personality is our method of dealing with our everyday life activities. It encompasses all our experiences, our pain and our peace and it is unique. People categorise us by our personality, they say, 'he is meticulous', meaning that he pays attention to detail, or 'she is shy', meaning that she does not mix and is quiet and reserved. Hence our personality is also how others see us and identify us. It is also by definition a method of behaviour classification. If you are meticulous, that is how you behave; if you are shy, that too is a method of behaviour, but behaviour in response to what? In response to a problem is the answer. Our lives are orchestrated by a continuous series of problems which must be solved before we move on to the next one. If you solve a problem successfully, you will remember it and use that method again in the future.

Successful problem solving develops particular behaviour in different people. However, although we use different methods of behaviour for different situations, gradually, and in very definite circumstances, each individual will polarise towards his/her favourite problem solving behaviour. What causes this to happen? Quite simply it is the inherent quality of a problem to cause us anxiety; the greater the anxiety, the greater the problem and the greater the problem, the more people revert to their favourite method of solving it. Therefore, if you are faced with the slight anxiety of meeting someone for the first time, you say very little to avoid making silly social mistakes – you are shy. When confronted with speaking to a group of people at a party, the anxiety you experience is even greater, so you do not speak to them at all but hide in another room — you are withdrawn. You are consciously aware this is happening, and in itself, as long as it does not actually interfere with your personal happiness and well being, it is not really a great problem.

However, if you develop this single favourite mode of dealing with anxiety to the point where it actually interferes with the smooth running of your daily life, you could have the makings of a mental illness. For example, two individuals are in a supermarket wishing to buy a tin of baked beans, and they are confronted with several alternative brands. The first individual selects the tin he wants by simply checking comparative prices, weights and brand names. However, the second individual cannot find the brand he usually has and cannot decide upon an alternative. The longer he takes trying to make the decision, the more anxious he feels, till in the end he makes no choice at all.

So far, one individual's selection and alternatives offer no problem, no threat and no anxiety, yet for the other, in exactly the same situation, the anxiety he experiences is so high that he behaves in a seemingly abnormal fashion. The more serious illness behaviours create an even more mystical shroud around the individual's life, because in an attempt to hide his failings, fears and anxieties from himself, he creates mental pictures to fill the gaps left by his own social incompetence. It then becomes almost impossible for him to distinguish between fact and reality. Sometimes it can take only the smallest of problems to push an already highly stressed individual into such a maladaptive situation; at other times it is a slow and insidious process which is almost impossible for the clinician to unravel.

Social incompetence is an inability to behave in a manner which maintains personal satisfaction in an acceptable way, making others avoid you

'How does psychiatry differ from psychology?'
Psychology is the study of normal human behaviour. It is necessary for psychiatric personnel to have an understanding of normal personal growth and behaviour if they are to understand the complexity of the psychiatric response. There are basically five major schools of thought related to why we behave the way we do (see below). The school of thought you agree with most will dictate what you feel is responsible for creating the expression of psychiatric illness.

Theories of the development of human behaviour

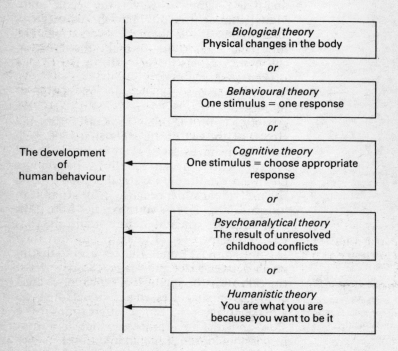

The development
of
human behaviour

Biological theory
Physical changes in the body

or

Behavioural theory
One stimulus = one response

or

Cognitive theory
One stimulus = choose appropriate
response

or

Psychoanalytical theory
The result of unresolved
childhood conflicts

or

Humanistic theory
You are what you are
because you want to be it

Final Comments

The psychiatric ward will probably be unlike anything you have encountered before. It may give you a little insight into some of the awful expressions of psychological distress and intellectual disorganisation that people are likely to experience when they are unable to solve their life problems successfully. Your job will be partly to try and use your own personal skills within the various care programmes provided to promote recovery, partly to make personal contact so that the patients feel able to vent their feelings in a safe and satisfactory way, but mainly to create an environment where they can regain social competence with dignity and confidence.

One final thought: the concept of 'cure' has a different significance in psychiatry. It can best be understood when considering a realistic definition of psychiatric nursing: to help a patient overcome those problems which inhibit his ability to lead a normal and purposeful life, or more often – when this is not possible – to help him come to terms with the effects of those problems and live his life with purpose and self-respect.

TEST YOURSELF

1 In what ways do psychiatric wards differ from their medical counterparts?

2 How does a psychiatric patient differ from you, yet why is he so much like you?

3 What is your role within the psychiatric ward?

4 Personality is an expression of behaviour. How is it involved in the production of a mental illness?

FURTHER READING

DARCY, P. T. 1984. *Theory and Practice of Psychiatric Care*, pp 10–27. London: Hodder and Stoughton.

IRVING, S. 1983. *Basic Psychiatric Nursing*, 3rd ed, pp 67–8. Philadelphia: W. B. Saunders and Co.

JUNGMAN, L. B. 1979. When your feelings get in the way. *American Journal of Nursing*, **79** (June): 1074–5.

2 Peter, who seems anxious

Peter is a married man of 24 with a good job, his own house, a little boy of 1½ years named Andrew, and a wife slightly older than he is, called Susan. Just recently he has been told that he is up for promotion and although everyone else is happy for him, Peter has been having doubts about his own ability.

Since he had the news, he has visited his GP on several occasions complaining of chest pains and difficulty with breathing. He has given up smoking and his social life has become non-existent. He is increasingly agitated around the house, often shouting at his son and refusing to go to work. His mother, who lives only a few streets away, has taken to visiting him every day, offering both advice and criticism and they have argued considerably about trivial matters.

His relationship with Susan is now 'tense', with no sexual activity at all, continuous arguments, and Susan threatening to leave him unless he 'grows up'. She is keen for him to accept the new post, as she wants him to succeed. She views his current behaviour as ridiculous, and tells him that he is making them both look silly in front of their friends and family.

Peter has always, by nature, been something of a worrier. He never makes big decisions without first consulting his wife, even though she may have little actual say in the matter. Before he was married, he relied heavily on his parents and in particular his mother for guidance and support. An intelligent and capable man in the abstract sense, his job is mostly concerned with computers and their operation. His promotion, however, involves meetings, business lunches, and a completely new set of responsibilities on top of his existing ones.

He has become restless, both at home and at work, biting his fingernails, eating very little and losing weight, finding it difficult to get to sleep at night and always wanting to talk into the early hours of the morning. He has only attended work once or twice each week for the past five weeks; although at present there is little threat to his job because of his absenteeism, he is worried that this may develop if he does not improve his attendance record.

His G.P. cannot find any physical dysfunction in either his respiratory or circulatory system though both are somewhat over-active with a B/P of 150/100. He had placed Peter on anxiolytic medication, Valium (Diazepam) 5mg three times daily and Mogadon (Nitrazepam) 10mg to help him sleep. After a few days, Peter refused to take them any more because he felt they might do him some harm and his wife thought that he should be able to manage without them anyway.

On his latest visit to the G.P., he was accompanied by Susan. She wanted the doctor to tell Peter that he was being foolish, that he should get back to work and resume his responsibilities as a husband and father. She described how at the weekend when out shopping with her, Peter had suddenly became panicky in the supermarket. His eyes bulged out of his head, he was sweating profusely, he rubbed the palms of his hands together continuously and did not appear to hear a word she said. She told him to pull himself together, but before she knew what was happening, he had fled from the store, knocking shopping trollies, display stands and even people out of the way. Two hours later she found him at his mother's house, crying, shouting, and gesticulating wildly with his hands. It took several hours to calm him down, and even longer to cajole him into returning home with her. She exclaimed to the doctor that she had simply had enough of this childishness and that if Peter was not 'sorted out' soon, she would leave him.

Peter said very little during the consultation; he kept wringing his hands, looking out of the window often and biting his lip. He fidgeted in his chair and generally looked very uncomfortable. When asked about the incident in the shop, he said that he had not meant to do it, but really could do nothing about it at the time. He was very apologetic. He did not seem to be able to comprehend what was happening to him and looked tired and a little unkempt. The G.P. had a few words of a supportive nature with him which he did not really hear and as he was about to leave, he started to complain once again of his chest pains. He refused to leave the surgery and started repeating that he was sorry, but he just could not do it. He was hyperventilating, flushed and sweating profusely. His eyes were fixed and staring with their pupils dilated.

The G.P. eventually calmed Peter down and felt, in view of the incapacitating nature of his expressed anxiety feelings, plus the dominant influence of his wife, that perhaps admission to a psychiatric unit might be the most immediate solution. Susan was horrified, but soon agreed when the situation was fully explained. The G.P. telephoned the unit and spoke to the psychiatrist on call who agreed to see Peter straight away, with a view to admitting him.

Explanatory note: most people who suffer from excessive anxiety reactions are usually treated within the community by their own G.P. A smaller number are seen through out-patient referrals to psychiatric clinics, but some, because of the extreme nature of the response, need to be brought into hospital. Hospitalisation often brings about even more stressful situations for the individual to deal with, not least of which is their eventual discharge.

Supportive care with anti-anxiety medication within his own environment is always the first choice because it enables the person the opportunity to actually come to terms with the situations creating the anxiety.

Hospitalisation, as in Peter's case, is often a last resort, used only because it creates a breathing space for all concerned, and enables the patient the opportunity to observe his life situation in a more objective fashion, as he is no longer actually involved in it.

ADMISSION TO THE WARD

When Peter came on the ward, having been seen by the psychiatrist, he appeared much calmer. In fact, once he had been told by the G.P. that he could come to the unit, there had been a remarkable change in him, and he seemed genuinely pleased to be here. His wife brought him in but soon left, saying she had to get back to Andrew. Peter was troubled by her departure, and watched anxiously as she disappeared through the doors.

NURSING CARE

Initial stages

The staff nurse who admitted him had several priorities. She needed to try to establish just how much his feelings of anxiety and panic affected his ability to carry out his life functions. She must discover just what it was that Peter hoped to achieve from being on the ward and what he thought would happen to him while here. She had to settle him onto the ward as quickly as possible so that his anxiety would not be heightened by his new surroundings, but he also required time and space to feel his way into the ward in his own way. She had to make a reasonable assessment of his immediate care situation and then spend the next few days establishing a more continuous plan of action.

She kept him informed from the very beginning as to what it was she wanted to do and why, and approximately how long it might take. Attempting to keep her voice calm and relaxed, she described the nursing role she would adopt with him, allowing him the opportunity to express his feelings and vent those areas of concern and confusion that he did not currently understand fully. In this way he could begin to relieve this emotional tension and help her construct a picture of his difficulties.

NURSING CARE

Observations

The nurse's immediate observations of him were divided into three main functional areas: psychological, sociological and physiological.

Psychological
1 Very restless, continuously shifting in his seat, standing up and walking around.
2 Appears agitated, asks for continuous clarification of statements made, seems anxious, gives curt replies at times, continually wringing his hands.
3 Does not appear to be able to concentrate on the subject being discussed, has to be allowed to verbalise in a rather rambling fashion.
4 Is absent minded, keeps forgetting where things are, particularly his personal belongings.
5 Keeps making statements like, 'I feel so helpless' and 'What am I to do?'

Sociological

1 Far too over talkative – will not listen to what is being said, keeps interrupting, all his conversation is centred solely around himself and his family.
2 Makes no real attempt at two way communication.
3 Smells of perspiration.

Physiological

1 Frequent visits to the toilet to micturate.
2 Dry mouth, asked for cold drinks several times.
3 Complains of feeling physically weak.
4 Said he had diarrhoea and feels a little nauseous.
5 Appears flushed, sweating heavily.
6 Respiration 35 / pulse 100 / BP 150/100.
7 Complains of feeling tense.
8 Looks a little unkempt, especially his hair, and he had also cut himself shaving.

NURSING CARE

Assessment

Most of Peter's behaviour was consistent with a severe anxiety reaction. He was not in any state to actively participate in serious clinical activity and he would need time to adjust to the ward environment. The nursing diagnosis was based on the most obvious and debilitating of Peter's current behaviour difficulties.

1 Feels uncomfortable in his new surroundings and as a consequence fails to communicate any real information about his feelings.
2 Is physically agitated and restless, which does not allow him the opportunity to relax at all – probably creates initial sleeping difficulties.
3 Because he cannot concentrate properly, he

becomes more distressed and frustrated with himself.

Objectives

The nurse's immediate requirements are to begin trying to establish a good working relationship with Peter so that he feels safe in her presence, able to speak to her on equal terms, and senses that she would accept him for what he was without making value judgements concerning his behaviour.

She also needs to involve him in the construction of his own initial behavioural objectives but without overwhelming him with decision making difficulties. He must see how his behaviour has altered, and by what means, so that he can more effectively cope without the guidance of the nurse if it appears once again at a future time. They mutually agreed on the following initial objectives for Peter. He would:

1 Try and remain seated within the day area for periods of half an hour at a time.
2 Construct a list of items which were uppermost in his mind at the moment.
3 Discuss the contents of his list at six o'clock that evening.
4 Get to know one other patient on the ward.

Intervention

This would be the plan of action for the first day, for review in the morning.

1 To give a minimum of 10 minutes to Peter each hour until after the evening meal and then to talk to him at six o'clock about his list for one hour.
2 To monitor his anxiety-promoted behavi-

our for areas of actual dysfunction, including sleep pattern.

3 Try to establish the exact nature of Peter's anxiety expression and the overt behaviour behind it.

4 Monitor the effects of presented anxiolytic medication.

5 Acknowledge him without approach at every opportunity, i.e. show that you have noticed Peter by nodding or smiling at him even though you do not actually go to speak with him. It is not always possible to spend a continuous period of time with him, so in this way you demonstrate that he is not forgotten nor is he being ignored simply because you are not with him. He will begin to develop confidence in you which hopefully will grow as more contact is made.

THE FIRST DAY

Peter settled into the day area. He had a bath and wandered around the ward. At discussion times he had to be reminded that he was trying to keep seated and relaxed. He had no lunch or evening meal and drank endless cups of tea. He got into conversation with a group of patients but soon left, although he did manage to hold a brief interaction with a female patient who appeared to show a sympathetic approach towards him.

The nurse while conversing with him had to try to blend sympathy and genuine concern with optimism and empathy. Empathising with a patient, or showing that you can see why a patient feels the way he does without actually feeling it yourself, is one of the more humanising factors within the patient/nurse relationship. She had to begin to create a degree of self-confidence in Peter so that he could explore his own life problems later in his stay. For now it was simply important that he felt safe to talk freely.

Explanatory note: the nurse must achieve a) the relief of the patient's emotional tension, b) a situation in which the patient can explore what he believes to be the causes of his behaviour and c) an outline, from the patient, of alternative methods of behaviour that will solve these problems more successfully. This simple counselling technique is sometimes called psychiatric first aid and although its stages can be used in quick succession where necessary, the first few days of hospitalisation are usually taken up with simply allowing the patient the opportunity to air his thoughts and feelings.

In this way, the nurse begins to form a clearer picture of what it is the patient is trying to achieve. It also enables her to clarify her own role within that activity.

Almost as expected, Peter had great difficulty achieving his own objectives. He produced only a scanty list of problems, and failed to remain seated unless in the company of someone else for more than a few minutes at a time. He talked constantly and became quite agitated and distressed when he could not say what was really on his mind. He sought out staff throughout the evening and the nurse had to seek some help from another member of her team as no member of his primary team was on duty during the evening and she could not keep up with Peter's conversation after a while. His wife did not visit in the evening, nor did she telephone, much to Peter's annoyance. He was afraid that something might have happened to her and insisted on calling her. She hung up on him.

The primary team is a method of nursing where ward staff are split into working teams responsible for particular groups of patients on the ward

Despite night sedation in the form of 10mg of Nitrazepam and a further 10mg two hours later, several hot drinks and supportive talks in darkened areas of the ward, Peter did not get to sleep till 0230 hours and then very restlessly. The night staff were concerned about the effects of Peter's wife's apparent rejection of him and his emotional responses to the whole situation. Anxiety is often accompanied by feelings of profound sadness or depression (see Chapter 3), and these contribute towards a general decline in the patient's ability to collect his thoughts in a linear and objective pattern.

Anxiety and the individual's day

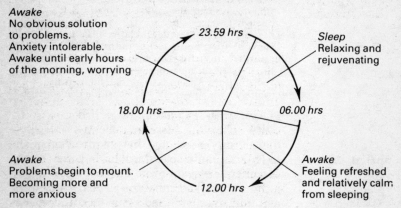

Awake
No obvious solution
to problems.
Anxiety intolerable.
Awake until early hours
of the morning, worrying

23.59 hrs

Sleep
Relaxing and
rejuvenating

18.00 hrs

06.00 hrs

Awake
Problems begin to mount.
Becoming more and
more anxious

12.00 hrs

Awake
Feeling refreshed
and relatively calm
from sleeping

Cognitive activities are the process of thinking, which is often called *cognition*

Explanatory note: because of the nature of anxiety, patients find great difficulty in getting to sleep at night. The reason for this can be understood when the patient's day is taken as a whole. In the morning, despite perhaps sleeping restlessly, he feels relatively relaxed. The brain has had an opportunity to rest from its cognitive activities and life does not seem quite so daunting. As the day wears on, so the anxiety increases, as the lack of solutions to his problems has an effect on his worrying and apprehension. The greater the uncertainty, the greater the feelings of anxiety become. The patient will eventually get to sleep in the early hours of the morning, with night medication (Nitrazepam – Mogadon), plus considerable supportive interaction by the night nursing personnel, though it may not happen for several nights following admission. However, as the next day progresses, once again the same problems re-appear, once again without solutions, and the cycle continues.

PETER'S FIRST WEEK

It became fairly obvious that Peter is not as acutely pre-occupied with his symptoms as had been originally thought. He responds well to being involved in his own care programme and works well within the nursing sessions. With the aid of his primary nurse, he con-

The primary nurse is the leader of the primary team, or group of nurses on a ward, usually a qualified nurse or senior learner

structs a hierarchy of his problems as he perceives them, and they use these as a basis for conversation. As a consequence, he takes part in off-ward occupational therapy which acts as a diversional tool, and concentrates more effectively on real problem solving situations. He begins to be a little more positive towards both his work and family environments. His apparent day dreaming and absorption in his chest pain disappear completely. Because his day is broken up with different activities, both clinical and recreational, he is less immersed in the apparent helplessness of his own personal situation. He remains over talkative, looks anxious and distressed at times, but the nausea and diarrhoea have disappeared. By the end of his first week, his sleep pattern is beginning to return to what it was before he was admitted, although it is still a long way from his own normal.

NURSING CARE

Rehabilitation

Unlike some patients suffering from the effects of severe anxiety, Peter will probably be in hospital for only a few weeks. During that time, both he and the nurse have several major objectives to achieve.

The nurse must continue to try and build upon the patient/nurse relationship, thus giving Peter confidence to speak about those areas of concern that cause him so much difficulty. She endeavours to teach him to find elements about himself that are positive and commendable, so that he does not see himself as a failure. She tries to show him how to identify the signs of his own anxiety, so that he becomes aware of himself and his possible problem areas. She also teaches him to relax, using relaxation therapy. This is a simple systematic method of self induced relaxation. It is often achieved initially by responding to the commands of the nurse, or to a pre-recorded audio cassette, with the objective that eventually the cassette will no longer be needed and Peter will be able to relax when confronted by his feelings of anxiety. She must support him and show that she cares for him as an individual by having him make as many decisions, good or bad, about himself as possible and reinforcing them at all times.

Peter's main objective, apart from learning how to recognise his own feelings of anxiety and relax accordingly, is to rest. If he is resting, there will be less anxiety to interfere with his decision making process and he has a better chance of being accurate in his problem tackling. He must consider, through discussion and counselling, just what he really wants out of life, and to come to terms with his own limitations in a more personal and acceptable way.

Whether the nursing staff actually play any part in reconciling Peter with his wife will depend on two factors. Firstly, they need to know what his feelings towards her really are and whether or not he wants others to be involved. Secondly, if the nurses do become involved, they must know to what extent they are to encourage him. They would have to work in conjunction with the other professionals helping Peter and their role might be that of counsellor when he vents his ideas and feelings on them, discussing alternatives and possibilities for his relationship with his wife. The couple might even meet in the company of one of the nursing staff to try to iron out their differences with the nurse acting in the guise of a 'chairman'. Whatever the role adopted by the nurse, she must at all times resist the temptation to give advice. Peter must find ways himself of coming to terms with his relationship, and he can only do that if he is guided through problem tackling techniques. If the nurse gives advice, it may be faulty; even if it is correct, the next time a crisis occurs, Peter will not have the experience of problem tackling to fall back on and will seek out the nurse once again to 'solve' the problem. He must find out what his wife truly expects of him so that they can come to some mutually agreed contract, and this may be achieved through family therapy under the guidance of either a clinical psychologist or the psychiatrist.

<table>
<tr><td>

NURSING
CARE

</td><td>

Planning discharge

</td></tr>
</table>

Much of what happens to Peter will dictate his actual discharge, both in terms of time and context. No two patients are the same despite their similarities in terms of clinical diagnosis. How they respond to that diagnosis, as individuals, will determine what happens when they are discharged. In Peter's case he felt that he probably would be capable of the promotion due to him, but with support. This he hoped to receive from his wife, although it would be technically variable, and more significantly from regular visits from his community psychiatric nurse and by joining the self help group, Neurotics Anonymous. The group will provide him with an obvious arena in which to vent his feelings about himself and his environment without having to resort to forms of avoidance behaviour once again. He would also have to keep taking a limited amount of Valium (Diazepam), but only until he felt he could manage without it. His prognosis depends on his willingness to use the counselling facilities available and his own real desire to succeed.

Evaluation

In all situations involving intervention by a nurse, it is of great importance that an appraisal be made of the effectiveness of the nurse's in-put. In Peter's case this would be done on a regular basis both formally at his care evaluation sessions and regularly on an informal basis by the nurse or nurses taking part in his care programme, both during and after each period of contact or intervention. Their effect upon him plays such a critical part in his recovery that it is necessary to monitor everything which they have done to bring about both positive and negative responses in him.

More specifically the development of the patient/nurse relationship requires careful evaluation to be used to its best effect. The degree of teaching, counselling and support may be dependent upon the time actually spent with Peter and this, in turn, could be influenced by the feelings the nurses have towards him. If they get on well with him, feel that they are achieving something positive with him and gaining some personal satisfaction from caring for him, they are likely to spend more time with him. If none of these elements are present they might spend less time with him or even unconsciously avoid his company except when the care plan actually called for it. Thus, in effect, the quality of the care he received would be greatly diminished. They need to identify such feelings of professional rejection in order to consciously overcome them and maintain full contact.

1   Outline the factors in Peter's situation that you feel were responsible for him being hospitalised. Having done so, rank them in order of influence.

2　The nurse's priority, when Peter was admitted, was to begin to establish a working rapport with him. State why this should be so important.

3　From the text of Peter's case, outline the major contribution made by the nurse in bringing about his eventual discharge.

FURTHER READING

BENDIX, T. 1982. *The Anxious Patient*. Edinburgh: Churchill Livingstone.

MADDISON, D. & KELTEHEAR, K. J. 1982. *Psychiatric Nursing*, 5th ed, pp 164–92. Edinburgh: Churchill Livingstone.

WATKINS, P. N. & GOODCHILD, J. L. 1980. *The Care of Distressed and Disturbed People*, pp 50–78. London: William Heinemann Medical Books Ltd.

3 Wendy, who is depressed

Wendy is a 38-year-old divorcee living alone in a rented two roomed flat, as her two children live with her ex-husband. She has not had a job for over a year and has little or no social life. On two separate occasions, once before her divorce four years ago, and once in the past six months, she has taken an overdose of sleeping tablets and been admitted for in-patient care to the psychiatric unit of her local general hospital.

As a result of her second admission, which had lasted for two months, she has been attending an out-patient clinic and receives supportive care visits from the community psychiatric nurse. She had been a member of a local after-care organisation designed to provide social activities and recreation for lonely people but failed to appear in the past few weeks.

One of the voluntary helpers was worried about Wendy as she had never really successfully contributed to the group, being always something of a loner and a worrier. She went to Wendy's flat but could get no reply and, fearing the worst, contacted both the police and Wendy's social worker. The police broke into the flat and found Wendy in her bedroom sitting up in bed, surrounded by what appeared to be all her personal belongings. She refused to speak to them, told the voluntary worker to go away and would only hold a very limited conversation with the social worker.

She was tense, irritable and appeared very sad. Her only topics were her 'miserable life' and her total condemnation of her husband. She blamed him for her failure to get a job or a decent house, and for taking her children away from her. She denied taking any form of overdose, but was morose, lethargic and disinterested in her surroundings despite the fact that her front door had just been broken down.

Her flat was in disarray, with dirty linen, unwashed cooking utensils and empty cigarette packets scattered all around. She said she had not eaten for several days, but really did not care, and from her appearance it seemed as if she had neglected much of her personal hygiene. She said she did not care about herself.

Her social worker was troubled by the whole scene as when Wendy had been reasonably self supporting, she presented as a meticulous individual, always keen to portray the image of a caring, independent woman. He knew that she was prone to withdraw from company when her problems began to get worse and he also knew that she had never really got over the apparent shock of her husband leaving her.

On both occasions when she had taken overdoses, it was because she had felt that people were conspiring against her. Although she denied ever seriously wanting to take her own life, the mere fact that she had made the gesture suggested a severe maladaptive response to her life situation. Her social worker spent nearly two hours with her and eventually called for the community psychiatric nurse. Between them they felt it was impossible for Wendy to remain in her own home, alone and unattended, and in view of her history it might be best for her to be re-admitted. Wendy's initial response was to refuse but in such a manner as to indicate that she really wanted to be persuaded that she ought to go. The two health workers were determined that she make the decision herself, and eventually she agreed. The nurse telephoned the duty psychiatrist and explained the situation, and Wendy was taken to the psychiatric unit.

Explanatory note: people become depressed, or extremely sad, for a variety of reasons, which can be grouped under two basic headings:

1 As a result of grief or loss
2 In response to continuous and often unwarranted feelings of guilt or unworthiness

These two groups present in different ways and it would be wrong to suppose that there is one classic picture of a person who is depressed. However, one factor inherent in the presentation of both types is the problem of self-harm. Where the individual has a previous history of such behaviour, it is usually advisable to admit them into care, but not always. In Wendy's case there was no one to whom she could turn for support; no one who would be prepared to provide continuous companionship within her own environment. Above all else the health professionals involved adjudged the situation to be potentially dangerous and, in view of her apparent disregard for her own safety and self respect, hospitalisation seemed the best course of action. Had the home environment been different, she might well have stayed out of hospital and been visited by members of a crisis intervention team. This is a group of people made up of doctors, psychologists, social workers, and psychiatric nurses whose function is to counsel and support people in their own homes when they have reached a crisis point in their lives. The aim is to get them to solve the problem for themselves without the added difficulties of hospital admission.

ADMISSION TO THE WARD

On her arrival on the ward, Wendy spoke very little, and what she did say was monotoned and monosyllabic. She was shabbily dressed, appeared unconcerned about her surroundings, held her head in her hands and presented as a picture of extreme sadness. The admitting nurse did not force conversation upon her but instead showed her to her bedroom, and over a cup of tea, told Wendy a little of herself, her role and how she would be her particular nurse.

No attempt was made to force Wendy to do anything in particular and the nurse was careful not to make any statement which might denote a sign of impatience on her part. She kept her tone of voice sympathetic, but not patronising. Her two main aims at that time were to make a biopsychosocial evaluation of Wendy, thus correlating her response to her emotional reaction, and to start the patient/nurse relationship so that the admission would be as painless as possible.

Biopsychosocial refers to biological, psychological and sociological factors involved in an attempt to gain a total view of an individual

NURSING CARE

Observations

While the psychiatrist interviewed Wendy, the nurse took the opportunity to talk with both the social worker and the community psychiatric nurse. She made a written account of her immediate observations, dividing them into physical, psychological and sociological groups.

Physical

1   Looked miserable and sad.
2   Sallow complexion – red rings around her eyes.
3   Unkempt and untidy appearance.
4   Some evidence of psychomotor retardation.
5   Bad breath.
6   Complained of indigestion, and hinted at constipation.

Psychomotor retardation is the general slowing down of all physical activity caused by a slowness in the individual's thinking process

Psychological

1   Flattening of mood, expressing depressive and morbid thoughts.
2   Seemed generally disinterested, with short concentration span.

Flattening of mood means becoming increasingly sad with no variation in feelings

3 Some evidence of anxiety present – wringing hands when not holding head – biting nails.
4 Short tempered, thinks this is all a futile waste of time.
5 Bursts into tears at regular intervals.

Sociological
1 Did not wish to sit in the day area of the ward, nor have any contact with other patients. Expressed the desire to be left alone.
2 Blames her husband for making her feel this way, but does not wish to see him or hear from him. Did not mention her children.
3 Speech monotoned, monosyllabic at times and could be quite curt and abrasive in her manner.

This data, linked with that of the community health workers gave the nurse some indication of Wendy's response to her feeling of depression. The nurse would need to identify other possible maladaptive behaviour not immediately available, so that she could construct a better profile. This included information about:

1 Whether or not she was ruminating over suicide or self injury.
2 Her sleep pattern.
3 Dietary and elimination activities.
4 Her feelings towards her hospitalisation.
5 Her feelings towards her social environment.
6 What her expectations of life are.
7 How she felt she could be helped by the psychiatric team.

None of these elements would be observed during the initial stages of her admission and indeed the pyschiatrist's interview only shed some light on the suicidal potential. Wendy was deemed to be contemplating some form of suicidal activity, if only a gesture to prove her true helplessness. It was therefore decided that for the time being she should receive close contact care at all times with individual nurses having specific responsibility for being with her. Their role would be to strengthen the existing tenuous patient/nurse relationship, make Wendy feel safe in her new environment, generate data about her thoughts and feelings and provide company for Wendy even if no one actually spoke with her. In effect, they would be 'specialling' her, because at that moment in time she was something of an unknown entity and with a previous history of suicidal activity, none of the staff were prepared to take any risks with her personal safety.

Explanatory note: providing constant contact while nursing an actively suicidal patient such as Wendy is a particular skilled job. The nurse has several objectives and sometimes her loyalties to the patient and her professional code can be antagonistic. On the one hand she must try to make absolutely sure that the patient does not harm herself in any way, yet on the other hand she must allow the patient the space and freedom to express herself as best as possible. Ideally the nurse responsible for this special role should be an experienced one but even if not, she should not have any other current responsibilities which might distract her from the patient. Sitting quietly with the patient, even if you are not involved in conversation, can become both tiring and stressful, thus it is important that some regular rota system is adopted. As few nurses as possible should be used, so that the patient can identify and relate to the people involved in her care. The degree to which this is carried out and the time span it requires will be dictated by the nurses' joint evaluation of the patient's suicidal status and the degree of acceptance of her situation that she exhibits. Each individual patient must be treated in relation to their own unique response – there is no set time for this practice.

Unfortunately before any contingency plans could be brought into play, Wendy had forced the issue. In the split second between the doctor leaving her and the nurse taking her place, Wendy had smashed the window in her room and was furiously sawing at her wrists with a jagged piece of glass. The nurse had been nearby, but while her attention was taken momentarily by something else in the room, Wendy had acted. It appeared to be a spontaneous act, totally unplanned, but nevertheless a very strong indication of her psychological state.

Despite the apparent viciousness of the attack, Wendy did not really do much damage. The psychiatrist checked the injury and apart from it being dressed, no other care was necessary. More importantly, the nursing staff had to help Wendy learn something positive from her actions. It seemed to them that she had been seeking some sort of clarification that the seriousness of her feelings was appreciated by all involved. Therefore, it was important to clarify this point.

For the nurses present it was also necessary to evaluate the incident, its effects upon them and the resulting influence it might have upon their approach to Wendy. They must discuss what had happened in order not to feel guilty about Wendy's actions. They agreed that it would be impossible to be one hundred per cent certain that they could prohibit Wendy from acting in the same way once again. While remaining in close contact with Wendy and monitoring her personal safety, the nurses also need to behave in such a way as to ensure her personal integrity. They could not be seen to be making decisions for Wendy, nor could they allow her to carry through the decision to harm herself in any way. This dilemma was discussed fully by those nurses who would be caring for Wendy. The result was that they supported each other while evaluating their approach and this enabled them to pay more attention to their own actions, their observational activities, care objectives and their effects upon Wendy herself.

NURSING
CARE

Initial stages

Empathy is putting
yourself in the
psychological
position of another

A nurse stayed with Wendy. She tried to show empathy towards her. This humanising factor within any relationship enables one person to indicate to the other that they understand why they acted the way they did without actually having to experience the same emotional response themselves. Simple statements such as, 'You obviously feel deeply hurt by the whole experience', or 'You feel very deeply about this whole situation', are often useful in beginning the process. They show that the nurse cares and yet does not patronise. Above all else they are factual statements about a real and demonstrable emotional situation, and do not reflect criticism on the part of the nurse.

NURSING
CARE

Assessment

An assessment of Wendy's situation identified several care areas:

1 She was angry both with herself and her husband for her current feelings but blamed her husband for her actual situation.

2 She had become overwhelmingly sad about her life as she saw it and not having come to terms with her life style, saw no real future for herself.

3 She actually wanted someone to help her and indeed was anxious that she should be seen as being 'ill' enough to receive help.

4 She had neglected herself because she simply could not see the necessity of carrying out the activities of daily living. They had become meaningless.

Objectives

These had to reflect the immediate care needs to be effected, and as a consequence of Wendy's intentional self injury, they centred around her personal safety.

1　Was prepared to injure herself spontaneously, either as an attempt to gain help or as a demonstration of her helplessness.
2　Expressed feelings of hopelessness and anger towards herself and her husband which needed to be reconciled.

These areas were discussed with Wendy as it was important to involve her in the care process from the very beginning of her hospitalisation. It was felt that her immediate care objectives would be coming to terms in some shape or form with these two objectives of the nursing diagnosis.

Intervention

1　For an allocated nurse to remain with Wendy at all times.
2　To try to discuss the nursing diagnosis and to attempt to get her to make some form of statement about her hospitalisation.
3　To remain calm and sympathetic towards her without interfering in her own chain of thought.
4　Not to make any value statements about her actions and not to push her into making decisions about herself.
5　Not to reinforce the feelings of hopelessness she had about her life situation. This would be done by trying to distract her to identify positive things about herself as opposed to the negative ones she was currently concentrating upon.
6　To prevent any further attempt at self-injury.

The nursing staff also made a provisional list of positive features in Wendy's presentation. All too often only the negative, maladaptive features are considered and this produces a rather illness orientated picture of the patient. It is only through identifying good things in a person's life that growth and a return of self confidence can be achieved. The nurses will use their list as topics of conversation with her in an attempt to generate feelings of reassurance that everything was not as bad as she perceived it to be. They would also initiate the process of logical thinking and create an atmosphere in which real problem tackling could take place.

The psychiatrist elected to keep Wendy in as an informal patient as he could see no reason to place her on an observation section of the 1983 Mental Health Act. In effect had he done so, he would have limited her movements and been able to keep her in hospital had she wished to leave, but Wendy was quite prepared at this stage to remain in hospital. He prescribed Tryptizol (Amitriptyline) 25mg three times daily and Librium (Chlordiazepoxide) 10mg three times daily. Tryptizol is a tricyclic anti-depressant which has some sedating properties, and Librium is a minor tranquilliser or anxiolytic which will counter anxiety. He could have placed her on an anxiolytic tricyclic anti-depressant such as Sinequan (Doxepin) or Prothiaden (Dothiepin), but the anti-depressant effect of these is not as effective and Wendy was deemed to have a more than mild depression.

An anti-depressant is one of a group of drugs designed to lift the mood or feeling sense so that the individual can experience a full range of emotions

Unfortunately with these anti-depressants the actual therapeutic effect may appear anywhere up to 14–21 days after the initial dosage. Therefore intensive nursing care must be a formality with the depressed individual so that the drug has the chance to work properly. As many as 80 per cent of patients taking this form of medication respond favourably towards it.

FIRST
NIGHT

REM sleep or rapid eye movement sleep is a period during a normal sleep pattern when dreaming takes place

Wendy was very restless all night. She hardly slept at all and with no obvious sign of REM sleep. Most of her sleep came in the early hours of the morning. She had begun to talk to the night staff about her feelings but in no great depth. She was rather unapproachable and distant and as the nurses wanted her to make the initial verbal responses, long periods of silence were experienced. When she eventually awoke in the morning, she seemed a little more alert and responsive, even to the point of suggesting she have a bath. She refused breakfast. Her movements were slow and deliberate. She still seemed anxious, wringing her hands and keeping her head bowed, and did not have eye contact at any time.

Explanatory note: there are deemed to be two basic forms of depression – one neurotic or reactive, and the other psychotic or without an obvious cause. Most authorities, however, agree that both are precipitated by some change within the individual's environment and in most cases the patient is prone to responding in a depressive fashion. The two forms of depression differ in basic presentation in several ways, but the diurnal mood swing is a factor in both. Wendy is diagnosed as the reactive form and thus the actual process of care takes a different approach to that for a psychotic depression. The identification of the cause of her feelings is of paramount importance as is coming to terms with it. Because her personality remains relatively intact, she is better able than the psychotically depressed individual to cope with this process. She also has a much greater potential for real recovery.

FIRST WEEK

Several observational factors were satisfied during the initial week. Wendy presented with:

Physical
1   Initial insomnia often until two or three o'clock in the morning and then sleeping poorly.

Possible differences in presentation of psychotic and
neurotic depression

Psychotic Depression		Neurotic Depression
General mental function may be impaired, especially memory and concentration	1	General mental function usually unimpaired though may suffer effects of anxiety
May mistrust others and become irrationally suspicious of their intentions	2	Tends to blame others
May attempt to hide real emotions	3	Openly overreacts
Suicidal attempts often well planned	4	Suicidal attempts are usually spontaneous
Feels that either he or his environment has been unrealistically altered	5	Remains in contact with reality
May suffer auditory hallucinations	6	No real perceptual disturbance
Total loss of appetite	7	In some cases may actually experience an increase in appetite
Wakes between 2 and 4 am	8	Cannot get to sleep until 1 or 2 am
Feels relatively better in the evening	9	Feels relatively better in the morning
Has no real insight into his behaviour	10	Often understands what is happening though not necessarily why

2 Poor diet taken, only eating snacks, biscuits, etc.
3 Poor elimination pattern, was obviously constipated.
4 Poor physical activity, either seated all day or wandering around in her room on a constant treadwheel circuit.
5 Washing habits improved a little.

Psychological
1 Her mood began to lift a little with the intense contact with other people.
2 She began to consider her life situation and began to participate in the production of her own care objectives.

3 She identified areas of strength that she had, but refused to accept that life actually had anything to offer her.

4 Blamed her husband for everything.

5 Missed her children almost to the point of distraction. They became the one most talked about topic of conversation.

Sociological

1 Some limited response to other selected patients, but most verbal activity took place with assigned nurses.

2 Could not concentrate on diversional activities.

3 Remained difficult to talk to because she would not initiate conversation and because she found the silences in her interactions stressful.

Suicidal probability scale

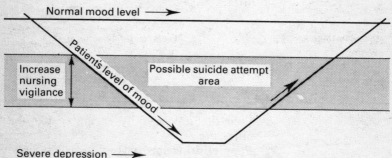

Explanatory note: the lifting of Wendy's mood, though a desired effect of care, is also one which produces another set of problems. She has made no further attempt at self-injury. Although not yet responding to the therapeutic effects of the anti-depressant medication, she was obviously benefiting from close contact and the freedom to ventilate her emotions. However, it often happens that as the mood begins to lift and the patient appears more cheerful, she is most at risk. It has to be remembered that she is still depressed and may well be capable of a self-injury attempt once again. The nurse must be particularly aware of this factor and keep as vigilant as possible in her care. The patient should not be left alone for long periods of time and should have no access to sharp objects or possible poor security areas, i.e. open staircases, tall buildings, main roads, etc. unless in the company of a nurse. She must be fully observed to have taken her prescribed medication, and not be hoarding it for a possible overdose. In doing all of this however the nurse still has to remain a therapeutic tool, a counsellor, a teacher and a friend.

A junior nurse learner might find it difficult to carry out all of these roles as they take considerable practise to perfect. It may be necessary to limit her personal target to maintaining a safe environment for Wendy whilst remaining as calm and approachable as possible. Indeed being approachable is the beginning point for some of the more advanced nursing techniques that Wendy will need if she is to recover. The nurse must also allow the patient to live with as much dignity as possible. This can often be achieved by inviting patients to make all the decisions, once fully discussed, in their own care programme.

NURSING CARE

Evaluation

Wendy's physical observations were consistent with the type of response that would be expected from an individual with psycho-motor retardation. As the psychological processes slow down, so do the physical ones. Although the constipation could be easily dealt with by a moderate increase in exercise and a modified diet, the sleep disturbance was more worrying. The nursing staff felt that as Wendy's mental state improved so too would her physical competence. It was necessary, however, to concentrate some attention on her personal hygiene and her approach to her evening activities. They encouraged her to take an interest in her appearance, discussed cosmetics and toiletries with her at set times during the day, and complimented her whenever she made even slight progress.

Rehabilitation

During the evening, a programme was produced that would involve Wendy in a set of activities eventually culminating in her retiring to bed with a warm drink. A nurse accompanies her during the final stages of the programme and ensures that conversation before retiring would be about happy, cheerful subjects of a positive and rewarding nature. Hopefully this will reinforce a feeling of well-being generated by the care programme and place Wendy in a better frame of mind to sleep. The night staff were included in the production of the programme as they will be responsible for its final implementation, and Wendy herself was involved in its production also in an attempt to interest her more in her own care programme.

The nurses' priority would be to gradually withdraw supervision of Wendy as she became more equipped psychologically to deal with her own emotional response. An accurate record of her behaviour was necessary because only by comparing her presentation regularly could the primary nurse actually make decisions about her own interventions. She needs to encourage Wendy to look at herself positively and uses active listening techniques to make her increase her verbalisations. The increase in the depth of the patient/nurse relationship constitutes the basis upon which this will be achieved.

The need for counselling, teaching and friendship stems from a mutual understanding of each other's requirements of the relationship and the nurse must promote true problem tackling by Wendy. The nurse might employ relaxation therapy, social skills, activities and personal assertiveness training to increase Wendy's awareness of herself. Experimental activities, such as role play,

Role play, psychodrama, music and art therapy are all forms of projective techniques used to help the individual examine their own feelings and come to terms with them. These techniques are usually carried out by experienced nurses

psychodrama, music and art therapy may be used to generate ideas about dealing with her emotional responses, and recreational and diversional therapies may play a great part in maintaining a balance in her hospital life. Too much work and not enough play may well make Wendy revert to her original behaviour.

Approaches used to increase Wendy's recovery

Social skills therapy

Role play

Recreational therapy

Psychodrama

Diversional therapy

Wendy

Music therapy

Relaxation therapy

Art therapy

Obviously Wendy needed to feel that her hospitalisation served a purpose, otherwise the necessity to demonstrate her feelings of frustration may well have provoked a further self-injury situation. However, she also had to begin the process of rebuilding her life. She would accomplish this by:

1 Giving a clear picture of what she wanted to do with her life once she had come to terms with the fact that she might not have any real contact with her children.
2 Identifying the feelings of depression and sadness before they became intolerable so

that she could do something to counteract them.

3 Giving herself the confidence to develop her life so that she receives some degree of pleasure from it.

4 Increasing her own sense of self identity.

5 Learning to communicate her true feelings to people without resorting to maladaptive behaviour.

6 Above all else, accepting the need for personal change.

Wendy's period in hospital would be dictated by her ability to achieve some of these objectives and to begin to recognise the others. The need to seek re-employment and construct a social life would be her basic practical objectives on discharge. With any luck a link with her children might be established, so that she might feel a greater responsibility towards them.

TEST YOURSELF

1 Identify the kind of behaviour that Wendy had adopted when she was admitted to the psychiatric ward.

2 At what period of time in Wendy's progression through her condition was she most at risk from self-harm? How could the nurse prepare herself for this eventuality?

3 What do you consider to be the nurse's role while nursing someone like Wendy who apparently has no desire to carry on living and yet may well have a perfectly good life could they but see it?

FURTHER READING

WATTS, C. 1980. *Defeating Depression*. Wellingborough: Thorsons Publishers Ltd.

WHITE, C. L. 1978. Nurse counselling with a depressed patient. *American Journal of Nursing*, **78** (March): 436–9.

DUBREE, M. & VOGELPOHL, R. 1980. When hope dies – so might the patient. *American Journal of Nursing*, **80** (November): 2046–9.

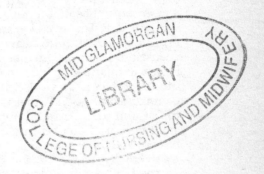

4

Alan, who is sometimes aggressive and violent

HISTORY

Alan has been in hospital for the last 10 days. He is 27, married with no children and works as a builder in a local firm. He demanded admission to hospital following an interview with his G.P. For several years Alan has been drinking alcohol quite heavily. He has been accused by various members of his wife's family of mistreating her and recently has had minor problems at work with his boss. He complained to his G.P. that things had got on top of him, that he could not cope any more and that if he didn't get into hospital quickly, he could not be accountable for his actions. He was verbally aggressive and insulting to the doctor, but later denied any of this.

ADMISSION TO THE WARD

At his admission interview with his psychiatrist, he displayed obvious signs of drinking and afterwards had been quite abusive towards the ward staff. When he had had time to cool off, and the effects of alcohol had diminished somewhat, the psychiatrist spoke to him again and it was agreed that he would have to establish for himself just what his priorities for admission should be. He also signed an in-patient contract that he would not drink alcohol while under hospital care. He was apologetic and appeared to be extremely frank and honest about himself, but the psychiatrist felt this was a façade.

For the first few days he appeared to be the ideal patient. He always seemed ready to discuss himself, his problems as he saw them and became involved in therapeutic activities designed to establish the nature of his personal difficulties.

On the fourth day, however, at a meeting of his primary nursing team, it became evident that he had been telling different members of staff totally conflicting stories. He had manipulated the team into several difficult situations which they had found almost impossible to cope with effectively. What became obvious was that, although he had said many things, he had not actually told them anything. There was some evidence that he had been drinking alcohol and also that he had struck his wife when she had visited. Neither of these two facts could be proven because he flatly refused to discuss them with anyone. The female members of the team found him quite charming as a person although they were suspicious of his motives, while the male members found him quarrelsome and surly. They found it difficult to make a positive statement about his initial few days without disagreeing with each other.

NURSING CARE

Observations

They listed the data that they had gathered about him.

Physical
There was no obvious problem with sleep, elimination, appetite, personal hygiene, etc., and he was in good physical condition – probably as a result of his work.

Psychological
These observations were more difficult to tabulate because much of the psychological

nature of any of Alan's presentations had to come from his own verbal responses, and there were so many inconsistences in his interviews that several different pictures materialised. The team agreed on the following:

1 He appeared to be suspicious of other peoples' motives for wanting to establish a working, professional relationship with him.

2 Pretended to give information about himself, but invariably the data was false or incomplete. He changed his story almost like a guilty man in a criminal proceeding.

3 He was rash in his praise, always wanting to please and became agitated if it failed to have the desired effect.

4 He was always defending his own actions.

5 He was very confident that his own observations about himself were correct. Often these would be quite derogatory, yet he took great pride in seeming to be critical and self analysing.

6 Despite being caught out with the discrepancies in his interviews, he never seemed to learn from his errors and would contrive to spin a web of intrigue around himself.

7 He was somewhat irresponsible, making improper suggestions to female patients and staff alike, and making statements that were totally out of keeping with his environment and situation, e.g. 'Let's all go out and have a great big party in the boozer; that'll do you more good than all these drugs they keep giving you.'

8 He was impulsive in that he would never sit and think a problem through but seemed to say the first thing that came into his head.

9 At the slightest hint of disagreement with him from any source, he would sulk and become moody and a little withdrawn.

Sociological

1 He did not appear to get on well with the male ward staff and had not participated as expected with his male psychiatrist. When asked about this, he denied this was the case and re-directed the conversation away from the subject.

2 He had made no relationship of any significance with any other patient.

3 He was intolerant of the views of others even if they were the same as those he professed himself in earlier conversations. It was almost as if he was looking for an argument.

4 He seemed to use others rather than enjoy them for their company.

5 Although not a statement about him, but rather about his effect on others, it was noted that one or two patients actually avoided him and seemed to be a little frightened of him.

NURSING CARE

Assessment

With all this information, it should have been easy to produce a tangible assessment of Alan that could be discussed openly with him and used as the basis for his period in hospital. Unfortunately, the vast majority of it was the observational material of the nurses and not from Alan and it was clear that he would object to large portions of it. The team decided to look at the positive aspects that Alan presented and use them as the basis of their presentation to him. It was felt that any real assessment of him that did not involve him would be unacceptable. Besides which they still did not really know what it was that Alan actually wanted. They needed to get at the heart of his requested admission. They agreed on the following nursing diagnoses:

1 Has made positive steps, through hospitalisation, to explore the problems he has and
   come to some workable solution for them.
2 Tends to become agitated when in the
   company of male staff who try to establish
   a working, professional relationship with
   him.

In view of Alan's approach to the different
members of the team, the second diagnosis
was carefully worded, but was still something
of a challenging statement.

Surprisingly enough, when Alan was presented with two diagnoses, he was in total
agreement. The first he simply accepted, the
second he was prepared to discuss at length,
stating that he preferred the company of
women, men were rather jealous of him and
this irritated him a little, for which he was
sorry. He felt it easier to talk to women because they seemed to understand him better.

Once again he said very little, although it
was becoming clear that he felt threatened by
the male members of staff. They were the ones
who asked him to question his behaviour the
most and thus appeared to be the stimulus that
produced the active response of aggression.

| NURSING CARE | ## Objectives |

Once again these were difficult to formulate,
especially as the member of the team responsible for preparing the work with Alan was a
male nurse. In view of Alan's limited insight
into the nature of his responses, it was agreed
that a compromise set of objectives could be
reached. Although they would not reflect any
real progress on his part, at least it would be a
step in the right direction for Alan.

1 Alan will identify those elements in himself which he feels to be his good points.

2 Alan will keep a written record of the times during the day when he feels agitated or angry. This will be discussed at regular intervals during each day, preferably as close to the incident as possible.

Explanatory note: it is unusual for people to be admitted to hospital in the way that Alan was. Many people actually request admission, but usually there is some positive evidence that hospitalisation will benefit them in some way. The major concern regarding Alan was essentially his alcohol consumption as opposed to his rather immature and explosive nature. A medical clinician would regard him as a psychopathic individual, or a personality disorder. This is usually a person who has an incomplete development of all facets of their personality making them insensitive to others, egotistical, rebellious, and at times anti-social. They have poor judgement and fail to learn from their mistakes. Because they do not adjust correctly to the social setting, they become easily frustrated and in the same way that a small child expects instant reward or response from its parents, so the psychopath expects to get what he wants without waiting for it. Indeed he often cannot see any reason for doing anything to get the reward, hence he often comes into contact with the police. As a result of the increase in frustration he feels towards the lack of response from those about him, he is more prone to becoming aggressive. This is the only way he has left to express his feelings. The alcohol in Alan's case is deemed to be a secondary problem exacerbated by his personality, and although his reaction to its withdrawal seems to reflect minimal levels of dependence, it may create still further problems of frustration for him. Other psychopaths may use sexual deviancy or drugs in the same way as Alan uses alcohol, as an escape.

Egotistical means thinking only of oneself

NURSING
CARE

Intervention

The team's major concern was to help Alan develop some insight into his own behaviour in an environment which was constant and secure. Every attempt had to be made to ensure that he did not perceive people being critical of him or making value judgements about his behaviour. There was also the necessity of involving his wife in the activity of care. However, due to his increasing aggression towards her, it was decided that she should be considered at a later stage in the care programme. The following items were those isolated by the team as their priorities:

Nursing response
Keep alert
Do not over-react
towards him
Speak quietly
Remain calm
Reward him if he
responds
Do not challenge
him
Do not leave him
Imagine how he
feels
Avoid physical
contact
Summon
assistance as soon
as possible if you
consider Alan to be
physically
threatening

**Modelling
technique is** an
approach used by
experienced nurses
which helps the
individual identify
and use the more
effective behaviour
of others

1 To establish through observation a base line of Alan's behaviour, identifying any elements which might constitute a pattern, trigger or cue to his agitation.

2 To compare their observations with his own record so that they could gauge the level of his insight.

3 To discuss his behaviour with him, using role play, psychodrama and modelling techniques, whenever the opportunity arose and to find alternative methods of behaviour.

4 To maintain a calm and consistent environment. This would include following a set policy towards him to ensure that he did not manipulate one member of the team to favour him where others had refused.

5 To use different methods of rewarding his positive behaviour and determine which produces the best response.

6 Avoid challenging him openly.

They also drew up a policy for the team outlining their own selected response towards him. This included:

Nursing response
Do not physically
restrain him on
your own
Call for assistance
of senior nurse
Pinion arms to side
from behind if
possible

1 Not over-reacting towards him should he become abusive.

2 Try to be aware of your own effect upon him.

3 Try to put yourself in his position to get some insight into the way he feels and see how you might respond in his position.

4 If he becomes physically violent towards

Hold arms and legs at joints
Lower him to the floor if possible
Lie across his hips and abdomen
Do not punch or slap in retaliation
Stay calm and do not provoke him
When possible, move him to a quieter environment
Once decision to restrain is made, act quickly and decisively

you, 'remain calm', do not retaliate, call for assistance.

5 Should the necessity arise that he needs restraining, this should be done effectively but with the minimum of force, the objective being safe and effective control for all concerned.

6 All aggressive or violent incidents to be discussed fully with all nursing staff concerned to explore their feelings towards the situation.

Explanatory note: there are many forms of aggression. We are all capable of it and in fact it is a natural way of venting our frustration. Hurling verbal abuse at the inept referee of a football match has almost become a hobby for some people in the UK and technically speaking is socially acceptable within the right social setting, i.e. the football ground. However, it would be totally unacceptable if the same supporters harassed the referee after the game, eventually punching and kicking him outside the ground. In other words, aggression has to fit the bill. Most drivers have the occasional word of wisdom for the other motorist, but only the real psychopath would actually carry out his threats. In Alan's case mild aggressive undertones have been exhibited in his response to his clinical environment. No one is really sure how he will respond if the team actually present him with a clear picture of his behaviour, and it is necessary to plan for all contingencies. The aim of any plan, however, would be to prevent violence from occurring; once violence has broken out, the aim is to stop it as quickly and as safely as possible.

Modes of aggression

Indirect (passive) aggression	Verbal (direct)	Direct
Being late	Arguing	Physical control
Forgetting names	Verbal abuse	Combativeness
Misunderstanding	Shouting	Fighting
Yawning	Swearing	Homicide
Refusing to speak	Demanding	Rape
Sulking	Blaming others	Suicide
Refusing to learn	Belligerence	Spitting

The medical staff had also been considering Alan's presentation and had decided that some form of medication might help his feelings of alcohol withdrawal. True, he had not appeared to experience severe symptoms but the increase in his agitation suggested that it was not easy for him. His psychiatrist had already prescribed Heminevrin (Chlormethiazole) 2 caps (192mg each), four times daily, reducing by one capsule each day. This drug has both a sedative and hypnotic effect, but is particularly useful for controlling alcohol withdrawal symptoms, those of delerium tremors (DTs). The usual dose for this condition is three capsules, four times daily, but Alan's condition did not warrant such a high dose.

However, when it was suggested that this medication might aid him in his alcohol withdrawal, he became extremely agitated, banging on the desk top, shouting and gesticulating at the psychiatrist. Although in the face of this verbal abuse the doctor remained calm and tried to reason with him, it had little effect and eventually Alan stormed out of the office threatening 'to do something serious' to anyone who tried to stop him from doing what he wanted. He left the ward, and as an informal patient, this was entirely his prerogative. A member of the nursing staff followed to see that he was all right, and returned later after having been verbally assaulted in the patients' canteen.

A hurried conference with all concerned showed that many had been surprised at the spontaneity of Alan's response and the nature of his aggression. The ward itself had been reasonably clear when the incident occurred but several patients had been upset and required support and reassurance.

One or two of the nursing staff felt apprehensive about Alan, and the psychiatrist admitted that he thought Alan was going to hit him during the interview. The staff supported each other, and talked through their policy in an attempt to approach the incident objectively. When Alan eventually returned to the ward, it would not be advisable to try to punish him in some way for his behaviour. He needed to examine his response in the company of a calm, rational individual and the nurse could not be that individual if she felt resentment towards him for making her feel frightened.

Possible causes of aggressive behaviour

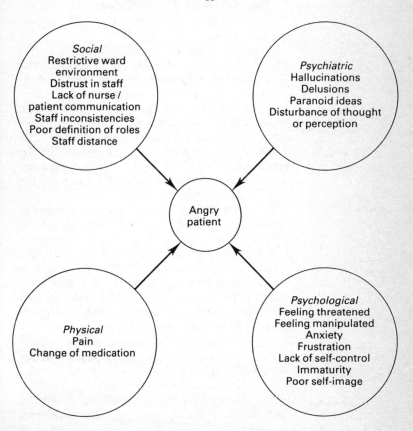

Social
Restrictive ward environment
Distrust in staff
Lack of nurse / patient communication
Staff inconsistencies
Poor definition of roles
Staff distance

Psychiatric
Hallucinations
Delusions
Paranoid ideas
Disturbance of thought or perception

Angry patient

Physical
Pain
Change of medication

Psychological
Feeling threatened
Feeling manipulated
Anxiety
Frustration
Lack of self-control
Immaturity
Poor self-image

Delusion is a false belief which cannot be shifted by logical argument and does not have to conform with sociocultural 'norms'

Hallucination is a false perception which has no external stimulus. It may affect any of the five senses

Paranoid thoughts involve the false belief that others wish to do you harm resulting in abnormal levels of suspicion

Disorientation is an inability to place oneself correctly in time or place or recognise others for who they really are

Explanatory note: in the same way that we are all capable of some form of violence, so too any psychiatric patient may become aggressive. The psychopath, such as Alan, uses violence as a method of getting his own way, while other patients' motives may actually be a misconceived self defence, stimulated by such problems as delusions, hallucinations, paranoid thoughts and levels of confusion and disorientation. The psychiatric patient as a whole is probably more prone to violence in any of its forms because of the distortion of his environment or the motives of those within it. In many cases, this can only be combated effectively by trying to find out what the patient sees and thinks. In this way, the nurse can begin to piece together a picture of how the patient feels. Although she may never fully achieve this, by at least starting the activity she will humanise her approach to the patient and hopefully reduce the amount of conflicting stimuli she offers him.

When Alan did reappear on the ward, he had calmed down considerably. He was apologetic and stated that he was prepared to 'go along' with anything that was suggested. The team felt that this was yet another example of him deflecting his responsibility for both his own actions and his own decisions. However, he avoided contact with the nursing staff for the remainder of the day, and it was deemed unwise to confront him with his behaviour the next day.

For the next week Alan's behaviour was the same. One minute he would be charming and helpful, the next shouting abuse at those around him and storming angrily from the ward. He never remained on the ward following these incidents and managed to avoid discussing them on his return. The team felt that they were getting nowhere with his care and reviewed their approach to him.

NURSING CARE

Evaluation

The team asked themselves the following questions:

1   Had Alan attempted to identify elements in his behaviour which were desirable or undesirable?
2   Did he have any understanding at all of his need for such explosive outbursts?
3   Had he stated what he really wanted from hospitalisation?
4   Had he really given up drinking for the time being?
5   Did he really want to change in any way?

The answer to all these was 'No'. Neither medical nor nursing staff could really identify a justifiable reason for Alan remaining in hospital under these circumstances. When this was put to him, he became, as expected, verbally abusive, stating that now the hospital had let him down, that they were turning him away, and if anything should happen to him, it would be their fault. Further, he refused to consider discharge.

The team used the approach they had agreed upon, remaining calm, not threatening him, and keeping a low profile as he vented his feelings. They did attempt to elicit some positive statement about his hospitalisation from him, but once again, following a further verbal tirade, he strode from the ward.

| NURSING CARE | ## Planning discharge |

They discussed what could be offered to him, and it was very little. Most psychopaths have very little room for change. After all, he had become the way he was in the same way that anyone else develops into the person they are. How could they treat him for being himself? He had consistently failed to show any real commitment to change, and was at times a liability, both to staff and patients. They were concerned that should he be discharged, his

**Alcoholics
Anonymous is** a
self help voluntary
organisation
providing support
for alcoholics who
wish to stop
drinking

wife might take the brunt of his anger, and,
besides, without planning his discharge, how
could they offer him any support? They still
had not identified the true nature of his alcohol problem, and Alcoholics Anonymous were
unlikely to consider him.

The initiative was taken from them however, because Alan, refusing to be discharged
by the hospital, discharged himself the next
day, still angry, still blaming the hospital for
his own behaviour. The Social Services and his
G.P. were informed so that they could take any
necessary follow-up steps. The team held a
meeting to consider their own feelings and to
gain something positive from the encounter
with him. All felt that for one reason or
another, Alan would probably be re-admitted
at some future date. They knew that little
could be done to help him within the traditional psychiatric setting where the true
criteria for admission is the motivation on the
part of the patient who wants to improve his
ability to lead a satisfactory life. The social
control had to come from Alan, not from the
nursing staff, and he had failed to achieve this
successfully. They also knew that, in time, he
might improve his behaviour simply because
he will become a little older and a little wiser,
but he has just as much chance of breaking the
law, and being sent to prison, or becoming a
chronic alcoholic with all the problems inherent in that condition.

In response to their own input, they questioned whether their approach had been correct? Had they asked too much of Alan? Had
they formulated the correct intervention? Had
their policy for aggressive behaviour been
appropriate? They satisfied themselves that
they had been realistic in the expectations and
their attempts to achieve them. Furthermore,
despite Alan's discharge, they felt that by the
use of regular meetings to discuss their feel-

ings towards him, they had been able to co-ordinate their intervention and provide each other with the material support vital in such a potentially intimidating situation.

TEST YOURSELF

1 Describe the features in Alan's presentation consistent with those of the psychopath.

2 What are the objectives of care for the psychopath in a hospital setting?

3 What measures did the nursing team adopt in an attempt to combat Alan's aggression?

FURTHER READING

BARASH, D. A. 1984. Defusing the violent patient before he explodes. *R.N.* **47**, 3: 34–7.
BURROWS, R. 1984. Nurses and violence. *Nursing Times*, **80**, 4: 56–8.
GRANT, M. & GRIMMER, P. (Eds.) 1979. *Alcoholism in Perspective*. London: Croom Helm.
IRVING, S. 1983. Sociopathic reactions to stress. In S. Irving, *Basic Psychiatric Nursing*, 3rd ed: 251–89. Philadelphia: W. B. Saunders Co.

5 Diana, whose behaviour is designed to gain attention

Diana is described by her friends as an out-going, carefree individual who is good at her studies and enjoys life to the full. Her supervisor of her drama studies course at university considers her overemotional, far too subjective in her application to research and prone to dramatise the least little incident.

These two conflicting opinions about the same person presented something of a problem for the primary nurse responsible for Diana's care. Two days previously she had been admitted informally on the recommendation of the medical officer at her university. He had been asked to see her because she complained of losing her voice. He could find no obvious physical abnormality, and she was not experiencing any pain.

On several occasions in the past, he had seen her in the medical centre and on each visit she had complained of symptoms for which he could find no obvious somatic signs. He had counselled her about this, yet despite her apparent intention to seek treatment, she was not unduly concerned by her ailments. He discussed this with her supervisor and discovered that her visits often coincided with either the presentation of difficult projects or examinations. He decided to talk to her about this but had not got round to it. Thus, when he discovered her to be complaining yet again from some incapacitating condition, he questioned her boyfriend about her immediate academic activities. He learned that she was about to make a series of important presentations in two weeks' time, but that she felt that she had no problems with them.

Diana dismissed the doctor's suggestion that her condition might be precipitated by stress and stated flatly, in a polite whisper, that she could not speak properly.

<table>
<tr><td>

ADMISSION TO THE WARD

</td><td>

With her studies reaching a critical stage, the doctor decided that some form of psychiatric investigation was a priority. Surprisingly enough, he had little difficulty persuading Diana that such a course of action would be in her best interests. The psychiatrist who admitted her described her behaviour as being like that of a person, 'soldiering on despite great tragedy'. She was accompanied by a whole group of people, all fretting and trying to help in some way. Her boyfriend was concerned that she was being admitted to a psychiatric ward, and asked if she could have a single room as she was 'not like the other patients'. He would not enlarge on this statement, and had indeed been told not to worry by Diana herself, who was still speaking in a whisper.

</td></tr>
</table>

Within hours of admission, her mother had arrived to be by her side, having travelled nearly 200 miles to do so. She fussed around her daughter, looking concerned whenever a nurse approached and demanding that something be done. Diana remained relatively calm and allowed her mother to control her immediate environment.

<table>
<tr><td>

NURSING CARE

</td><td>

Observations

Much of what her boyfriend and her mother said about Diana did not seem to ring true to the primary nurse. She was more inclined to

</td></tr>
</table>

Pre-morbid personality is the individual's personality or behaviour before they became unwell

favour the supervisor's assessment of Diana's pre-morbid personality. The impression gained by the primary team consisted of the following information:

1   Diana was an attractive 19-year-old who managed to manipulate others to get her own way, but did so in a charming way. It was almost as if those who cared for her felt it a privilege to help her out.

2   She helped around the ward, especially with the elderly patients and thrived on the praise given her by her relatives and friends alike.

3   When things did not go well for her, she would appear to be deeply distressed, yet at the same time stated that she understood, or that she would manage somehow. This display of apparent martyrdom left some of the nursing staff a little exasperated.

4   Apart from helping others on the ward, she did little for herself. She was keen to sit and discuss herself with the nursing staff. She seemed to be working hard to provide realistic data about herself that could be used to identify care objectives but resisted the temptation to actually formulate any idea as to why she had suffered a series of physically unrelated, and unproven conditions which had usually been associated with some forthcoming test of her ability.

On a biopsychosocial level, the team's observations followed a similar pattern.

Physical

Aphonia is the inability to speak

1   Complained of aphonia and spoke in a whisper.

2   No obvious physical difficulties noted.

3   Seems relaxed and content. The fact that she cannot speak properly does not appear

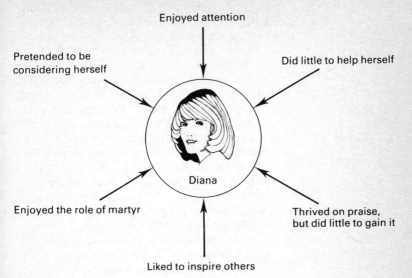

General initial impression of Diana

Enjoyed attention

Pretended to be considering herself

Did little to help herself

Diana

Enjoyed the role of martyr

Thrived on praise, but did little to gain it

Liked to inspire others

to worry her in the least ('la belle in-difference').

4   No complaints of pain.

Psychological

1   No amount of logical argument can sway her opinion about her voice – she remains convinced she is unable to speak properly.

2   Does not seem unduly concerned about her admission to a psychiatric ward.

3   Tends to over-react in potentially emotional situations. No tears, however.

4   Rather shallow in her actual emotional responses to realistic problems and the feelings of others.

5   Rather immature in her approach to her life situation.

Sociological

1   Appears to use her sexual attraction as a method of getting others to do things for her.

2   Although she calls him her boyfriend, she

actually treats him in a rather childish fashion. When together she is always snuggling up to him, touching him and teasing him. When apart, she never mentions him and does not appear to miss him. Moreover, he has stated that their relationship has never been very constructive as such and they spend very little time actually doing things together. He also stated that their sexual relationship had become non-existent with Diana becoming frigid.

3 Felt to be rather demanding and manipulative of the staff.

4 All conversations, held in a whisper, related to Diana and never ever included others unless they were introduced as subjects for discussion by the nurse.

5 The team generally felt that Diana was living a role that she had identified for herself which had cast her as the heroine in a tragic drama.

Explanatory note: Diana is suffering from the effects of a condition known as *conversion hysteria* and more specifically in her case, *hysterical aphonia* and *sexual dysfunction*. There are several forms of hysteria, but all are a form of behaviour which shifts the fear and anxiety of emotional conflicts into physical and mental symptoms. It is an unconscious process of which Diana is totally unaware, and to all intents and purposes she really cannot speak in anything but a whisper. She has nothing physically wrong with her. This form of somatic response

Different presentations of hysteria

Conversion hysteria	Dissociative hysteria	Associated syndromes
Disturbance of:	Fugue	Anorexia nervosa
Movement	Amnesia	(Nervous loss of weight)
Perception/senses	Forgetting things	Munchausen syndrome
Mood	Sleep walking	(Hospital addiction)
Seizures/fainting	Being accident prone	Gansar syndrome
Visceral sensations		(Approximate answer syndrome)
		Bulimia nervosa
		(Nervous overeating)

Splitting, dissociation, conversion are methods of unconsciously changing the reality of a situation so that the individual is unaware of their own failure (a Freudian concept)

can occur as paralysis, blindness, immobility, stomach cramps or any other physical symptom which is deemed appropriate. The individual is often unperturbed by them. The object of the mental defence mechanisms of splitting, dissociation and conversion, which produce the condition, is to protect the individual from the truth about his or her own failings. In Diana's case she feels that she cannot pass her forthcoming presentation, yet all around her are convinced of her talent and expect her to pass easily. The conflict here is simple to identify, though often it may not be. To protect her from failure, she has produced a somatic condition which gives her a legitimate excuse not to take part. In other words it distracts from the real problem of anxiety about failure, by giving those around her something more tangible to worry about. Other forms of hysteria include dissociative presentation such as amnesia, sleep walking and fugue state, while special related syndromes include anorexia nervosa and munchausen syndrome. Hysteria is unlike either psychosomatic conditions or malingering, but may be confused with them.

Hysterical reactions and alternative behaviours

Malingering	Psychosomatic disorders	Hypochondria	Conversion hysteria
not necessarily stress related	stress related	not necessarily stress related	stress related
conscious activity	unconscious activity	conscious and unconscious activity	unconscious activity
pretends to have a physical problem	does have a physical problem	misinterpretation of body sensations	thinks he has a physical problem
knows there is nothing wrong	may not realise that something is wrong	wants something to be wrong	thinks something is wrong
non-specific picture: problem often untestable, e.g. back pain	physical condition usually initiated by increase in stress, e.g. peptic ulcer	usually centres around problems of internal organs	unrealistic impression of debilitating complaint, e.g. total loss of feeling or movement in arms or legs

Assessment

Diana was considered to be strongly demanding attention and sympathy, not only from her friends and relatives but from the nursing team also. Her attempts to make people feel sorry for her, while trying to gain their respect by appearing to overcome her adversity, were a difficult subjective response for the team to overcome. Her primary gain through using this method of attention-seeking behaviour was to overcome the anxiety of her forthcoming examination; her secondary gain was to help her avoid failure. Her desire to escape anxiety in such a maladaptive fashion meant that she obviously had serious doubts about her own capability and was, therefore, not as confident and self assured as she would have others believe.

The team identified the following nursing diagnoses:

1 Is extremely anxious about forthcoming events and has lost her voice in an attempt to avoid trauma.
2 Uses her aphonia as a method of gaining sympathy and attention.

When these were discussed with Diana, she stated that she did not understand what they meant. She quoted her psychiatrist as saying that there was no physical problem, and the nurses telling her that she was 'pretending', yet she really could not speak. She became morose and looked lost and bewildered. However, the same ambivalence that she showed normally towards her aphonia, now reappeared towards the nursing diagnoses, and she seemed to accept them without much interest. This was unfortunate because the motivation to want to use normal or adaptive methods of coping with anxiety has to come from the individual, and in Diana's case, it obviously was not there.

The medical and psychological assessment of Diana's condition did not conflict with that of the nurses'. All representatives of the multidisciplinary team agreed that medical intervention for her would have to include some form of psychotherapy, probably abreaction, or drug induced hypnosis, in an attempt to get at the heart of her problem. The nursing intervention would have to complement this activity and create an environment in which Diana was re-motivated to want to regain her voice, and overcome the need to use hysterical symptoms as a method of avoiding anxiety. The team needed to identify positive aspects in Diana's presentation that they could use as the basis for this confidence building. Her care objectives and nursing intervention would have to reflect this intention.

Psychotherapy is conversation which involves listening to and talking to an individual in an attempt to help them understand and resolve their own problems

NURSING CARE

Objectives

The team wanted Diana to achieve quite a few things including gaining insight into her behaviour; knowledge of alternative methods of behaviour; and identification of her own internal conflict. It was agreed that the first steps in this process should be simple and effective. The following immediate care objectives were constructed with Diana taking an active part in their production:

1   She will discuss the possible psychological causes of aphonia with the primary nurse and make a positive statement concerning her own situation.
2   Will produce a list of behaviour she uses to elicit sympathy from others.

Diana regularly employed several tactics to avoid discussing her real anxieties and these too were discussed with her when the objectives were documented. In this way, the team hoped to create an environment in which Diana felt safe to discuss her real feelings and without fear of stimulating negative responses from the nurses.

Explanatory note: Diana is currently using her aphonia and emotional seduction, i.e. eliciting pity and sympathy from others, and to a lesser degree her sexual frigidity, to avoid talking about the real issue. Like many hysterically orientated individuals, this is often a successful ploy. In the clinical environment, however, the nurse must encourage the individuals to look at their problems and not at the anxiety they create. Many patients use styles of speech and linguistic codes to produce this avoidance effect. They employ such approaches as hostility or expressions of superiority towards the nurse, questioning the nurse's ability to do her job, circumlocution, i.e. pretending to answer questions while in fact talking about something completely different, superficiality, refusing to discuss anything in great depth, withdrawal, denial and intellectualisation. All of these approaches must be identified by the nurse if she can, so that she can begin to combat them effectively.

NURSING CARE

Intervention

To help Diana achieve her two objectives, the team had several alternatives at their disposal:

1 Promote growth of the patient/nurse relationship through active listening, warm and responsive interaction, allowing adequate time for her to reply to questions and being interested in her replies.
2 Not responding to her maladaptive behaviour in a way that would reward and reinforce it. This behaviour could not simply be ignored, but her whispering voice should not impede the flow of conversation and little reference to it should be made. Likewise when she tries to manipulate the conversation away from its dynamic course, she should be confronted with

Nursing response

Encourage role play activities

Do not let her change the topic of conversation

Help her to recognise feelings of anxiety

Encourage proper speaking habits

Promote nurse/patient relationship

Do not reinforce maladaptive behaviour

Teach her to relax

Encourage personal confidence

Help her to accept responsibility for her own behaviour

her behaviour, and the conversation allowed to continue as before. Any attempt on her part to try discussing these items at length, should be resisted.

3 Do not let her write things down but encourage a speech programme to help her to speak properly once again.

4 Help her to recognise the feelings of anxiety and the behaviour that they produce in her. Using an open ended questioning technique, the nurse should try to get Diana to talk about less threatening subjects and gradually turn the conversation to those producing conflict.

5 Supportive confrontation may help her to concentrate her thoughts on the subject matter. This should only be done if she attempts avoidance strategies however.

6 Teach her the process of relaxation. Despite her apparent calmness, which is only due to the presentation of her physical symptoms, she will experience considerable anxiety levels when discussing her real difficulties. Using relaxation therapy, the nurse can try to help Diana cope with some of the physical responses to the anxiety that she feels. It is important, however, that Diana be able to recognise the presence of anxiety related behaviour in order to begin using the technique to best effect.

7 Encourage the growth of her personal confidence through an examination of possible alternatives in behaviour. Allow her the opportunity to discuss ways in which she might behave that would be more suitable to real problem tackling, and create situations in which she could try them out.

8 Indicate to Diana that she must be responsible for the changes in her behaviour if she is to succeed in her attempts to overcome anxiety. If she is allowed to

escape this responsibility, then she will not have the necessary experience of problem solving to fall back on in future situations. As a consequence, she will only use those maladaptive responses she has found to be successful in the past.

9 Encourage role play situations to enable her to examine her own behaviour.

Throughout her initial hospitalisation period, Diana had received no form of medication. Often such individuals are given small doses of anxiolytics or minor tranquillisers such as Valium (Diazepam), but in her case this was not deemed necessary.

FIRST WEEK

She agreed to see her psychiatrist on a daily basis and they started to examine the root cause of her disability. Both medical and nursing staff kept each other informed of their relative progress so that they did not duplicate the therapy process. The main aim of the medical intervention was to establish the cause of Diana's conflict, while the aim of the nursing staff was to initiate a change in response to the anxiety it created. If the medical intervention was ineffective, they might use abreaction as a method of confronting the problem. This is a drug induced hypnosis, or twilight state, in which the patient is 'talked through' her internal conflicts, facing up to the realities of the anxiety responses and verbalising her feelings about them. Theoretically, once the individual has faced the problem successfully, the somatic symptoms should disappear because they are no longer required. In practice, however, the anxiety usually settles on yet another difficult area and a similar set of physical symptoms emerge. Abreaction is usually carried out by the psychiatrist accompanied by a nurse as it requires the intravenous injection of drugs to bring about the hypnotic state.

Explanatory note: not all forms of attention seeking behaviour are as obvious as hysteria, but when the individual's motives, personality and maturity are examined, there may be many similarities. Much is designed to stimulate concern in others through feigned helplessness, or the more overt window smashing, self abuse and absconding which have qualities of the dramatic that cannot be ignored. The nurse must try to remember that this type of behaviour is usually a maladaptive way of seeking comfort, and as such must not be reinforced but cannot be ignored. The patient must be aided to explore alternative methods of behaviour more appropriate to the situation and these instead must be rewarded so that they are perpetuated. The possible approaches that Diana's nursing team hope to adopt towards her may be used in the care of all recognised attention-seeking behaviour, the skill being in its recognition.

NURSING CARE

Implementation

During the next week, Diana was encouraged to talk about her problem, to identify areas of personal concern and examine the excessive emotional responses she makes towards others. The nursing staff tried to imagine themselves in her position to see how they might respond under such circumstances. This would hopefully give them an internal framework of reference from which to base their own reciprocal behaviour. They allowed her little leeway in conversation so that she was forced to concentrate on the more significant topics and they did not respond to her emotive pleas of helplessness whenever she felt cornered.

The staff counselled her about ways of tackling her anxiety, and experimented with alternative approaches. A record of events was kept and graphed so that Diana could visualise her progress. Therapeutic interactions were centred around one or two nurses only in an attempt to polarise objectives and reduce the possibility of repetition. She was encouraged to attend well supervised therapy sessions so that the focus of attention was taken away from herself for a while. Communication between herself and her university was maintained where possible so that she would not have the added problem of re-establishing links upon her discharge from hospital.

On the sixth day in hospital, she awoke to discover that her voice had returned. This 'miraculous' event coincided with the realisation of what she was doing, though at first she was reluctant to admit it.

NURSING CARE

Evaluation

Diana remained in hospital for a further four weeks. During that time she explored the possible causes of her condition and gained some awareness of her own behaviour and its motives. In such a short period of time, it was impossible for her to alter her approaches but at least she was offered the chance to examine her own response to anxiety and recognise its effect and then determine possible selective methods of dealing with it. Her care objectives were always achieved, as in most cases she created them and was aware of her own potential.

The influence of her protective mother was difficult to assess, although it was noticeable that she performed better without her presence. Her boyfriend was included in therapy sessions with the doctor and helped resolve some of her misconceptions about herself and the way others saw her. She agreed to visit her own doctor regularly to discuss her progress and the community psychiatric nurse followed up her return to the campus. It was hoped that her promising career would not be affected, but she had to be given support and guidance and the opportunity to discuss her real feelings whenever the need arose.

<table>
<tr><td>NURSING
CARE</td></tr>
</table>

Further evaluation

The nurses responsible for Diana's care programme maintained careful links with each other throughout her stay in hospital. This was necessary because they needed to gauge both the effectiveness of their own intervention and of Diana's involvement in her own progress. By evaluating their own input, at first on a daily basis and then gradually reducing to once per week, they were able to measure how much influence they were bringing to bear upon Diana's improvement and how much responsibility Diana was taking upon herself. They maintained two forms of evaluative procedure, one involving the nurses active in the care programme, and one also involving Diana. In this way they were able to clarify their own thoughts, present Diana with care continuity and provide a therapeutic arena for her to explore her own interpretation of her actions.

Once Diana had been discharged, the staff also carried out a retrospective nursing audit to evaluate the whole of the care programme, its effectiveness and suitability. It is important to establish which elements had been successful as well as those that had not been successful. In this way they could build on their knowledge for future care programmes by examining and using the successful ploys in their approach to other patients and avoiding the other actions that did not bring about the desired result. It is also possible to establish why each element in the programme had been successful or not.

The data were passed on to the community

psychiatric nurse who would be working with Diana on her return to University in the hope that she might also benefit from the team's evaluation findings.

Nursing evaluation of Diana's progress

Concurrent data	Daily nursing	Weekly nursing	Retrospective
Admission →	Diana's progress	→ Discharge	
gathering	evaluations	evaluations	nursing audit

TEST YOURSELF

1 Reviewing Diana's case, what would you identify as being the salient points in the hysterical person's pre-morbid personality, i.e. her personality before becoming ill?

2 What are the primary and secondary gains of people using attention seeking behaviour?

3 What approach would you adopt if faced by a person who continually sought your attention, but had no obvious reason for doing so?

4 How did the team intend to encourage Diana to use more acceptable methods of dealing with her anxiety response?

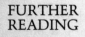

FURTHER READING

BILEY, F. & SAVAGE, S. 1984. Anorexia Nervosa. *Nursing Times* 80, 1, Aug: 28–32.

KONIKOW, N. S. 1983. Hysterical seizures or pseudoseizures. *Journal of Neurosurgical Nursing*, 15, 1, Feb: 22–6.

MERSKEY, H. 1979. *The Analysis of Hysteria.* London: Baillière Tindall.

WATKINS, P. N. & GOODCHILD, J. L. 1980. The management of attention seeking behaviour, in Unit four, Nursing the anxious patient. *The Care of Distressed and Disturbed People*: 62–7. London: Heinemann.

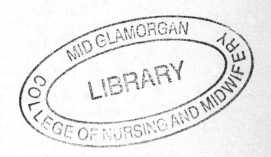

6 Grace, who is obsessional

Many, if not all of us, have certain rituals or routines which we carry out regularly. They may range from simply keeping one's hair in excellent condition to redecorating the whole house once each year. Some people have an immaculate garden, yet always look like a scarecrow in their dress; the filing system of some executives totally contradicts their pristine appearance. In short, to be meticulous about some aspects of our lives is quite common and perfectly healthy. However, in Grace's situation, her overt rituals have come to dominate her life to such an extent that they invade every facet of her existence. She has used them to combat her feelings of anxiety in an exclusive fashion and has to be admitted to a psychiatric ward.

Rituals mean repetitive formal behaviour which may be a cultural trait, but must be carried out for the individual to feel safe

Grace's father, a tough rigid man who had been in the Armed Forces all his working career, has recently died. He made Grace the executor of his will and although this did not entail a great deal of work, it had left her feeling confused and angry. She was an only child who had spent much of her early life travelling around the world on various postings with her parents. When her mother died, she and her father had drifted apart and, although they had never been particularly close, they had become virtual strangers. She went to university and despite a rather lonely academic existence, had done quite well. Now, at the age of 30, she was working as a librarian in a small county library and appeared reasonably content. Her colleagues described her as a serious individual, meticulous and scrupulously tidy. The perfectionist in her left her with few friends and her irritating habit of complaining of a series of minor illnesses exasperated those she did have. She was easily dominated, both in her work and limited social life, being quite timid and always appearing keen to please.

Her only real support came from her local church where she was an active member of several groups and committees. She was never really successful in these ventures but, being committed, was quite highly thought of. It was because of her friendship with the vicar's wife that she came to the attention of her G.P. Grace had become increasingly withdrawn, being more nervous than usual in the company of others and having great difficulty carrying out both her work and church activities effectively. Her skin and hair were noticeably in an appalling state, dry, flaky and in poor condition. She was increasingly late to every occasion and once had failed to open the library at all. When the vicar's wife visited Grace at home she was amazed to find that it was in an extremely untidy condition. Usually there would be nothing out of place, but it looked as though Grace had not tidied up for weeks. She appeared in her dressing gown and said that she was about to have a quick bath. Two hours later she was still in the bathroom, and no amount of cajoling could get her to come out. The vicar's wife eventually persuaded her to open the door and found that Grace had been scrubbing her hands, arms, legs and face with a small brush until they were red raw. When she eventually got out of the bath, saying how silly and ashamed she felt, she could not make up her mind which clothes to wear and it was evident that to get her to the doctor's surgery was going to take far more tolerance than was possessed even by the vicar's wife.

A home visit from the G.P. that evening was enough to convince him of the need for intervention of some description. Originally it was intended that Grace could stay at the vicarage but after three days she had made life intolerable for all concerned.

ADMISSION TO THE WARD

Grace had arrived in hospital wearing a nightdress and a housecoat. She refused to be brought in by car because she said it was unclean and an ambulance had been required for the one mile journey.

Her appearance was immediately noticeable. Although only 30 years old she should have been an attractive woman but she looked twice her age, her face and arms were red and swollen and her hair was brittle and dry without style or shape. She spoke in crisp tones and avoided eye contact. After politely refusing a cup of tea, she said she was not prepared to stay on the ward and wanted to go home. She was accompanied by the vicar's wife and another woman and they tried to persuade her to stay. The nurse, however, decided that it would be best to move Grace into a safe and comfortable area of the ward and discuss her reasons for wanting to leave. The two women left and Grace appeared a little more at ease.

The admission had taken nearly four hours, but eventually Grace agreed to stay, at least overnight. The nurse was concerned with the condition of Grace's arms and face but as she could see that Grace was embarrassed about them she avoided any direct comment. She talked openly about personal hygiene only when Grace brought the subject up.

Explanatory note: many patients are reluctant to be admitted to a psychiatric ward. They recognise the benefits that may be gained and often feel relieved to be amongst people who appear to understand and accept them. However, the feelings of failure consequent on such an action will often not allow them to take the admission easily. In Grace's case the situation was complicated by her awareness of her condition, both physical and psychological, and her apparent inability to do anything constructive about either. She was ashamed at having let herself get into such a state, having prided herself for years at being smart and respectable. She was unwilling to allow others to see her and the more this worried her, the more obvious and extreme her behaviour became. She had scrubbed herself for several hours in her own bath in an attempt, as it were, to wash away her guilt.

The nurse in such situations must try to show compassion and attempt to generate feelings of understanding. This may be achieved by listening intently to the individual, repeating phrases for clarification, and generally looking as if she really does care. She should avoid areas of obvious concern, and allow the individual the time and freedom to progress as they are able. At this stage, delicate topics should only be discussed fully if the individual mentions them. In this way the nurse is allowed into the individual's confidence and the patient/nurse relationship can begin to develop. If the individual detects signs of disgust or outrage in the nurse, the damage may be irreparable. The nurse must try to imagine how she might feel were the roles reversed. Admission for someone such as Grace must be carefully planned and painstakingly executed.

| NURSING CARE |

Initial stages

Grace had to be given as much support as possible. She needed to gain confidence on the ward, not to feel as if she was being punished in some way, and to begin to establish a place for herself within the care programme. The nursing team must establish the level of Grace's disability, the extent of her rituals, the nature of her feelings and their effects upon her. She was, therefore, allowed considerable freedom during the first few days so that these observations could be made and both positive as well as negative components of her presentation could be considered. She was permitted to carry out her rituals as long as they did not endanger her already scarred facial and arm

Do not overreact
towards her

Show no signs of
distaste or disgust

Encourage
awareness of
herself

Establish positive
elements in her
behaviour

Confront her with
her behaviour
sympathetically

Try to develop
trust between
patient and nurse

Listen intently to
what she has to say

Allow
patient/nurse
relationship to
develop

Observe ritualistic
behaviour to
establish level of
disability

Do not inhibit
ritualistic
behaviour unless it
becomes dangerous
for her

Ask her why she
needs to carry out
her rituals while
she is doing so

integument. However, she was counselled during these incidents and not simply left to function in a vacuum.

She persisted with between six and seven baths a day, using any number of towels and disposable wipes. She never got dressed and did not wear any makeup, although she combed her hair repeatedly. She said very little, appearing timid, shy, nervous and distracted when approached. Time was required for her to talk about herself, her father and her life as she saw it.

Observations

Physical

1 Integument in dry flaky condition, especially her legs.
2 Face and arms red and looking very sore. Not complaining of any discomfort.
3 Poor diet, poor eliminatory pattern. Refused to use the communal toilet facilities and requested a bed pan. This was given — followed by a bath.
4 Bathes six times minimum each day.
5 Cannot sleep until the early hours of the morning. Seems more refreshed but looks distressed.

Psychological

1 States that she realises all her rituals are silly, but when she tries to stop them, the urge to carry them out seems much stronger.
2 Complains of being aware of thinking obscene things, swear words, unpleasant thoughts about her sexuality, etc.
3 Says the rituals take her mind off these.
4 Feels she is unclean and could harm others in some way.
5 She is not sure but feels that in some manner she is responsible for her father's death.

6 Says that much of her dirt has stemmed from looking after the books in the library, which in turn she feels are filthy.

7 Feels guilty and says that God is punishing her.

Sociological

1 Does not wish to mix with others because (a) she will contaminate them, (b) they will despise her.

2 Cannot use communal facilities because they are dirty.

3 She says she has nothing personal against her fellow patients, this is just something to which she has a particular aversion.

Her willingness to talk about her condition and her feelings was achieved after several days of considered attention by the nurse. She had been seen on several occasions by her psychiatrist. No medication had been prescribed in an attempt not to cloud her presentation in any way. On the positive side several factors were evident:

1 She had some insight into the extent of her own behaviour including its consequences.

2 She wanted to overcome her situation.

3 She trusted several of the nurses enough to confide in them.

4 She had a relatively strong personality.

5 She was cared about by those people within the church circle who visited her regularly.

6 She still had both employment and accommodation.

These factors were important because it would be by accentuating them that the nursing team hopes to increase her sense of purpose and re-establish her sense of identity and self-esteem.

Behaviour rituals
Incessant handwashing
Continuous bathing
Over concerned with minute elements of personal hygiene

Explanatory note: most of us have tried to give something up in our lives, whether cigarettes, alcohol or just that extra cream cake. The most intriguing fact is

Scrubbing parts of body
Refusal of food prepared by others
Failure to dress
Over exaggerated daily routine
Will not use communal toiletry facilities
Pulling body hair out

In more severe cases:
Manual extraction of faeces
Self mutilation

Obsession is an idea, emotion or impulse which repeatedly forces its way into the individual's consciousness despite being unwelcome

that as soon as we try to give up, the need becomes greater and we may give in to temptation. We justify our actions by saying that it doesn't matter anyway, and besides we often enjoy what we are doing. The sense of guilt is short lived as a consequence. In Grace's case the situation is far more extreme. It is agreed that people such as Grace who experience guilt about their feelings become anxious to the point where they carry out simple rituals to distract themselves. In her case it could well be conflict caused by the strictness of her father and society's expectations of children towards their parents versus the need for a more flexible life and freedom from routine. As the guilt, here accentuated by the death of her father, becomes greater, so the rituals become more intrusive until eventually they dominate daily activities. At this point, they become obsessions and if resisted, just like the last cigarette, they become almost a necessity. Individuals may develop all sorts of behavioural rituals, but many are centred around dirt and cleanliness.

The thoughts experienced by Grace are called *compulsions*. They too become intrusive, are usually of a derogatory nature and can only be avoided if the obsessional rituals are carried out. Like Grace, most individuals realise the whole situation is of no purpose, yet they cannot resist its futility. If they do so, the anxiety and guilt are heightened and they may become suicidal.

NURSING CARE

Assessment

Grace readily agrees to be involved in the production of her own care even though she needs guidance and understanding. Her primary nurse explains in detail the observations she has made and Grace confirms or explains points as she goes along. It is important that the nurse does not assume Grace will place the same emphasis on each of the points that she has herself nor that she will draw the same clinical conclusion from the data. Empathy must be employed to mold the nurse's approach and to find mutual agreement or compromise where the two of them differ over the importance of the observational material. The following nursing diagnoses are agreed:

1   Grace's skin on her hands and face is red
    due to continuous rubbing and scrubbing
    during her numerous baths each day.
2   Is too involved with her rituals to spend
    time getting dressed and made up.
3   Cannot bring herself to mix informally
    with the other patients on her ward be-
    cause she feels she will contaminate them
    in some way.

NURSING
CARE

Objectives

It is very important that the same nurse tries to
establish just how much initial potential for
change Grace possesses. Grace must actually
agree to achieve any objective set, otherwise it
will be of no value constructing them. It is
intended to gradually reduce the time allowed
for each ritual while teaching Grace to use
thought stopping techniques and relaxation
therapy, so the objectives must reflect this
intention.

**Thought stopping
techniques** Each
time the obsession
appears the
individual is taught
to think of another
pleasant subject
until the obsession
ceases

1   By the end of the first week Grace will have
    reduced her baths to four a day, each of ¾
    hour duration. There is no actual mention
    of face or arm scrubbing as the reduction in
    time will begin to solve that problem; also
    if it were mentioned, it might actually
    increase her need to carry out the act.
2   By the end of the first week, Grace will
    dress each day, having selected her cloth-
    ing the night before. It will be necessary to
    increase gradually the number of clothes
    that she puts on each day, hopefully culmi-
    nating in full dressing by the end of the
    seven day period. At that time, the process
    can be consolidated and the act of using
    make-up started.
3   Grace will attend the weekly ward meeting
    of staff and patients but may be permitted
    to sit on the perimeter of the group. She

must be fully dressed. It is important that she begin to make contact once again, and that she be in a physical condition which will not attract attention from her fellow patients and thus reduce her already low self esteem.

Prior to intervention

Before discussing the nursing intervention, it is important to examine the complementary activities of the medical and non-medical members of the multi-disciplinary team. If Grace's anxiety and guilt levels are increased by the reduction of her ritual time, it may become necessary to prescribe anxiolytic medication. Likewise, she may become increasingly depressed at her failure to overcome what she already perceives to be a pointless and fatiguing obsession. This, plus the intrusive obscene thoughts she has, may result in a suicidal attempt. Careful monitoring of her mood will lead to prescribing anti-depressant medication, preferably of the Tricyclic type, for use if required.

Identifying the root cause of her problem may be the task both of the psychiatrist and of the psychologist using individual insight-directed psychotherapy. The occupational therapist will be brought in to fill Grace's spare time and try to divert her attention from her compulsions. He may also teach thought stopping techniques and eventually introduce Grace to a self awareness group or an assertiveness group.

Self awareness group is a therapy form designed to give the individual a greater understanding of themselves and the reasons why they behave as they do

Assertiveness group is a therapy form designed to increase the individuals' confidence in themselves and their social activities by practising social skills, e.g. eye contact, posture, dress and speech style

Intervention

It is likely that the intervention used with Grace will have to be limited by the primary team's commitments to the other patients in its care group. It would be unrealistic to identify pages of possible care that could never be implemented. This would produce frustration in the staff and resentment in Grace when she perceived she was not getting what was promised. The alternatives in caring for someone such as Grace will depend largely on the priority given to each problem area and the time, facilities and care already being utilised. The following are those items listed as meeting that criteria:

1. Employ a behaviour modification approach, using reward for success, that is, for reducing the time spent in baths and the frequency of bathing. Be firm with her about the availability of baths (such as the amount of time she can spend in them) but be kind in your approach so she does not see staff as threatening. Produce a time chart outlining when she can bathe, etc. Talk to her about it, get her to discuss it with the nurses. The time scale should be reduced every day. Congratulate her when she achieves the required daily reduction and remind her of the seven day target. Help her to rest.

2. Discuss clothing with her; the need for personal presentation and social acceptance; her decision making ability. Coach her to increase her commitment to dressing. Design a flow chart whereby she increases dressing activity and offer rewards when each daily target is achieved. If she does not achieve it, be firm with her without appearing demanding and redesign the chart highlighting the seven day objective.

3. Talk about her feelings of contamination, why they have suddenly occurred.

4. Produce with her a hierarchy of problems and tackle each one in ascending order of anxiety provocation. Once she is able to

contend with each problem area, move on to the next.

5 Introduce her, firmly but kindly, into the day area for an increasing time span. Take time not spent in bathing as a measure of time available. Do not force actual social contact with other patients unless she initiates it.

6 Teach relaxation techniques. Help her to identify an increase in anxiety and its effects upon her behaviour.

7 Teach thought stopping techniques. Each time the intrusive thoughts are present, make her talk about something pleasant – decide on the topic beforehand. If she is not in the company of someone knowledgeable, teach her to keep repeating a given word over and over again while trying to carry out some form of pre-arranged diversional activity.

Suicidal ruminations mean persistently thinking about suicide, suicidal activities and the necessity to avoid psychological pain through death

It will be vital to monitor Grace's level of motivation, her ability to achieve her objectives, etc. and to liase with the psychiatrist to measure how their two separate approaches are affecting her progress. Most importantly of all the nursing staff must try to identify any changes in the pattern of the ritual, as one ritual may be substituted for another, and also to detect possible suicidal ruminations.

Explanatory note: many individuals become so obsessional and compulsive that such approaches to their care are fruitless. Despite having an apparent insight into the behaviour, they are unable to identify its cause. It is essential that the team work together to produce a reversal in behaviour, and that all the effects coincide with the individual's actual needs.

Total approach to the care of the obsessional individual

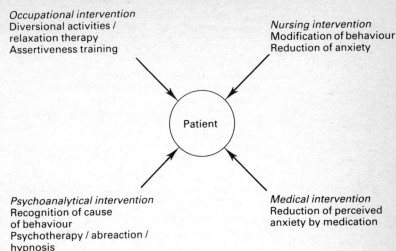

Occupational intervention
Diversional activities /
relaxation therapy
Assertiveness training

Nursing intervention
Modification of behaviour
Reduction of anxiety

Patient

Psychoanalytical intervention
Recognition of cause
of behaviour
Psychotherapy / abreaction /
hypnosis

Medical intervention
Reduction of perceived
anxiety by medication

NURSING CARE

Evaluation

Grace may spend several months in hospital and her progress will depend on the success she has in identifying the root cause of her behaviour. Her care objectives will have to follow a sequence that reduces maladaptive behaviour and increases adaptive. Several other facts will have to be considered both by her and the staff:

1 What are her social expectations and how does she view her work and personal environments?
2 Is she able to establish a workable and acceptable routine for herself?
3 Can she identify a realistic self image?
4 Does she wish to change her life style?
5 Can she talk openly about her relationship with others especially the opposite sex, marriage, etc.?

Her prognosis will depend largely on her.

Self image is a picture of oneself in relation to one's beliefs, attitudes and ideas in relation to our sociocultural surroundings

Care objectives for the obsessional individual

Increasing objectives	Decreasing objectives
time spent:	time spent:
talking to others	in seclusion
occupied constructively	carrying out rituals
venting feelings	reproaching oneself
examining causes of	listening to
guilt	compulsive thoughts
examining self image	feeling dirty or unclean
considering effects of	ignoring anxiety
anxiety	orientated feelings

```
                    ┌──────────────────────┐
              ┌────►│  Nursing objectives  │◄────┐
              │     └──────────────────────┘     │
              │     ┌──────────────────────┐     │
              └────►│  Patient objectives  │     │
                    └──────────────────────┘
```

Several further factors require consideration:

1 How long has she been using this maladaptive behaviour, and how much of it has evolved after modelling herself on her father?
2 How Grace feels about herself.
3 What motivation has she for change.
4 What effects will the nursing and medical intervention have upon her?

Throughout all of her time in hospital, she will need a mixture of kindness and firmness from the nurses while establishing a routine, the time and space to express her feelings and the opportunity to examine herself away from the pressures of her usual daily life. She must be encouraged to maintain the few links she has with people outside the hospital, so that when she does eventually return, she can hope to do so with some degree of dignity and self confidence.

TEST YOURSELF

1 What elements in Grace's personality could be said to have influenced the direction her maladaptive behaviour took?

2 What is the connection between obsessional rituals and compulsive thoughts?

3 Outline the basic approaches to care identified for the different groups within the multi-disciplinary team.

4 When nursing an individual such as Grace, what must be the objectives of the nursing intervention?

FURTHER READING

BROMLEY, S. 1983. Washing the pain away. *Nursing Mirror*, **156**, 1st June: 43–4.

FARRINGTON, A. 1983. Obsessive compulsive disorder. *Nursing Mirror*, **157**, 17 Aug. Mental Health Forum 8: vii–viii.

MERCER, S. 1984. Obsessive compulsive disorder. *Nursing Times*, **80**, 29 Aug: 34–7.

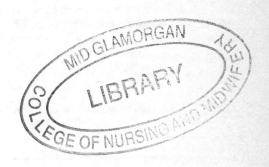

7 Isobel, who is highly suspicious and severely disturbed

Introduction

Each of the preceding chapters has dealt with behaviour which, in psychiatric terms, is regarded as being neurotic by nature. In each case, it has affected only certain areas of the individual's personality leaving other parts intact, much of the general mental function uninhibited if a little restricted, with often considerable insight on the part of the individual concerned. However, a large proportion of the people admitted to psychiatric wards suffer from a more severe group of behavioural problems which are collectively called a psychosis.

Psychosis is a group of severely disruptive conditions which affect all parts of the individual's personality including social contact, perception, emotion, language and thought

Contrasts in behaviour between the psychotic and neurotic presentation

Psychotic behaviour	Neurotic behaviour
All elements of personality involved	Only elements of personality involved
Loss of contact with reality	Contact with reality maintained
No obvious single cause	Often as a result of stress
Behaviour may be totally unpredictable	Behaviour often an exaggeration of normal responses
Behaviour not consistent with pre-morbid personality	Behaviour consistent with pre-morbid personality
Little, if any, insight	High degree of insight, to the behaviour if not the cause

From the point of view of medical diagnosis, they include the various presentations of schizophrenia, mania and psychotic depressions, and their consequences for the individual concerned are often quite dramatic. The role of the nurse is also different; as the behaviour exhibited by the severely disturbed is more dramatic, the objective is to provide reality orientation rather than seeking the elusive cause of the problem.

Reality orientation is a therapy technique designed to help individuals place themselves correctly in time and space

HISTORY

Isobel is 44 years old, married with two teenage children. She is a housewife who regrets never returning to her job as a teacher after her children were born. Her husband is a civil servant, and the family lead a relatively uneventful life style. On two separate occasions in the past, once for four weeks and once for two and a half months, she was admitted to a psychiatric ward. On the first occasion she was 36 years old and had to be formally admitted under an observation section of the old 1959 Mental Health Act. The second time, two years later, she agreed to be admitted, but again had to be transferred to a formal section while in hospital because she intended to leave against medical advice. For the last six years, she has been attending regular outpatient appointments, and has been visited fortnightly by the community psychiatric nurse who administered injections of depot medication to help maintain her in the community. She has managed to lead a perfectly healthy life since her last admission and the care team were pleased with her performance.

Recently, however, her relationships with her children had become more demanding. They were approaching their tricky adolescent period, and her husband was less than supportive in her bid to cope with the added stress. As a consequence of this, the familiar pattern of

Depot medication involves drugs, administered intramuscularly, with anti-psychotic and tranquillising properties. They are released into the blood stream over an average period of two weeks providing a constant mood and removing the necessity for oral medication.

behaviour that had led to her previous crises began to reappear. She was far more rigid in her approach to her family, intolerant of the children's attempts to establish themselves as individuals, and withdrew from any real communication with her husband. She felt increasingly suspicious of his actions, and threatened outside of her own home. She suspected that people were discussing her in public, criticising her behaviour and watching her continuously to find fault with her. She refused to answer the door to callers, convinced they intended her harm. She firmly believed people to be hostile towards her, and acted in defence of these beliefs by avoiding them at all costs. When the community nurse called, she could get no reply; when the children returned from school, they discovered that Isobel had barricaded herself in the house and refused them entry.

She threw milk bottles out of the bedroom window at passersby in the street, shouting abuse at them for alleged crimes they intended to commit against her. When her husband returned from work, he was no more successful in gaining entry to his home. No amount of persuasion would convince her that she was in the wrong; in fact, no real dialogue was possible with her because she flatly refused to talk to anyone. The police and her social workers were both called in to help. They too had little success, and although her husband gave his permission for the police to forcibly enter the house, it was decided that the G.P. should be called first in a last attempt to cajole Isobel into letting them enter peaceably.

Eventually, however, the police had to break into the house, and Isobel retreated to the bathroom. She spoke to the doctor and her husband through the locked door, but was still convinced that her life was in jeopardy, and shouted at them continuously. It was agreed she should be re-admitted to a psychiatric ward. As she had no intention of going voluntarily, and as she was considered by all present to be a threat both to herself and others, it was necessary to place her on a formal section. She was eventually taken to hospital, after much unpleasantness, under Section 2 of the 1983 Mental Health Act.

Factors which might have influenced Isobel's use of psychotic behaviour

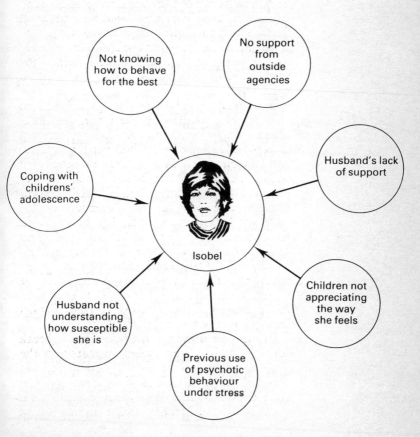

Explanatory note: in 1982 and 1983, changes in the Mental Health Act revised much of the previous legislation. Isobel was admitted on a section designed for assessment, possibly to be followed by treatment, for a duration of up to 28 days. Although such admissions cause extra stress for all concerned, they are often the only way that the individual in need of care actually comes into contact with the facilities and resources available to them.

ADMISSION TO THE WARD

The application for admission under Section 2 had been made by the social worker who accompanied Isobel, her husband and two police officers to the ward. As the section requires the recommendation of two registered medical practitioners, the consultant psychiatrist had visited Isobel's home. In separate interviews with the G.P., they had both agreed to her admission. Previous admission data had been found by the nursing staff, and along with the preliminary information from the psychiatrist's domiciliary visit helped to produce an idea of how Isobel might behave. It was important that not too many preconceived ideas were created as the approach towards Isobel by the admitting nurse ought to be spontaneous, caring and warm.

Isobel was obviously frightened and unhappy about her admission. She was given a booklet explaining her rights as a patient admitted under section, and her right of appeal was carefully explained by the admitting nurse. She appeared ambivalent to this event. She did not want her husband to leave her side, yet said some unpleasant things to him about getting her into 'such a place as this'. She refused to look around the ward though it was felt she should explore her new surroundings. Her room was not to her liking, and she wanted the door left open at all times. She questioned everyone about their intentions, sought clarification of every statement made towards her, and often attached the wrong meaning to simple events. Everything seemed to have particular significance for her, and she was convinced that she was not being told the truth. She said very little and weighed every sentence carefully before she spoke. She sat curled up in a chair in her room and became agitated if people entered her personal space.

<table>
<tr><td>

NURSING CARE

</td><td>

Observations

Isobel exhibited a considerable amount of observable behaviour, but little could be verified because of her unwillingness to communicate verbally.

</td></tr>
</table>

Physical
1 Poor attention to personal hygiene, being also rather scruffily dressed.
2 Her husband stated that she had eaten very little recently, was sleeping badly, often up all night, and that she seemed lethargic.

Psychological
1 She was convinced that her life was under threat and spoke occasionally of 'them'. She would not say who 'they' were, but smiled ironically and said she understood everything.
2 Her sentences were broken up, often disjointed with a strange use of associated words, saying such things as, 'So this is a hospital/life and death/death by murder/murderer in a prison cell/the cell is the basis of life/I am not pregnant, why am I in hospital?' This loose association was sometimes difficult to follow.

Auditory hallucinations are the hearing of voices which are not actually present. Usually the voices are speaking either about or to the individual concerned

3 She appeared to be listening for the slightest noise, though it was not possible to tell at that time if she was actually experiencing auditory hallucinations.
4 Emotionally she seemed rather flat, with little facial expression, yet she was de-

finitely frightened by her experiences.

5 Was suspicious of all around her, questioning their motives.

Sociological

1 Would not initiate any form of conversation.

2 Even after several hours she had made no attempt to mix with others on the ward, who were busying themselves getting ready for bed.

3 Was abrasive in her manner towards the nursing staff on the one hand, and condescending on the other.

4 She did not offer aggression in a physical sense, but was abusive from time to time, especially towards her husband.

NURSING CARE

Assessment

It was obvious that Isobel would need time to settle onto the ward, and the data gathered on her would need clarifying and expanding. However, she required immediate nursing intervention based on the early nursing diagnosis that she felt physically threatened, both by her environment and the people in it, and that she had no insight at all into the cause of these feelings.

The nursing staff tried to be very positive in their approach to her, using simple statements and unambiguous phrases. Non-verbal communication had to complement exactly what was being said. They attempted to listen very carefully to anything she said in return. No attempt was made to force her into doing anything she did not want to, and they did not discuss items of obvious concern. Any mention of suspicious ideas or thoughts were not disagreed with even if they were obviously ill founded, but neither were they reinforced by being avoided or by being deeply questioned.

Nursing response
Do not force her to make decisions
Non-verbal communication should not conflict with speech
Do everything you say you intend to
Be positive in your actions
Use simple unambiguous statements towards her
Listen carefully to

what she says
Be obvious in your actions
Do not reinforce suspicious ideas but do not disagree with them either – discuss if possible
Monitor initial effects of medication
Allow her to find her way around the ward

The psychiatrist prescribed Chlorpromazine (Largactil) 150mg three times daily with Dalmane (Flurazepam) 30mg at night should she request it. The night staff were unsure about whether she would take the medication in tablet form and were given permission to use Chlorpromazine syrup if it were easier. As it was, Isobel eventually agreed to the Chlorpromazine after it had been carefully explained to her, which took nearly an hour's intermittent work on the part of two separate nurses.

ISOBEL'S FIRST NIGHT

Delusional ideations are a whole series of ideas and beliefs which stem from an original delusion and which consequently are untrue

Isobel did not sleep at all until 0430 hours. She refused night medication, and the night staff could see no real reason for trying to persuade her to take it. She spent most of the time in her room in the company of a nurse, but did explore the geography of the ward from time to time. The content of her speech became more and more disrupted, she voiced real delusional ideations about 'them' (coming to get her, to kill her) and was convinced that the nurses were in on the plot. Despite this, she was incongruously pleasant for the most part towards the night staff. Her thoughts, when voiced, were disordered, and she had difficulty keeping to the point. On two or three occasions, she was found hiding in her room; on another she was heard shouting at someone, though on investigation, she was found to be alone. She slept restlessly till 0645, when she got up and demanded to go home. The night staff spoke to her at length, and although she was quite adamant that she wanted to leave, she would not explain why. She accepted that she was not allowed to leave the ward, but seemed to feel that this was all part of the plot to get her.

Different presentations of the schizophrenic individual

Schizophrenic reactions to stress	Presentation
Simple (disorganised)	Lacking in drive and will power Avoids contact with others Intolerant of others/hypochondriacal Social deterioration/personality decline
Paranoid	Feels persecuted but protests innocence loudly Emotionally unresponsive Hears voices (hallucinations) Remains socially aware
Catatonic	Unceasing activity (violent, destructive) or Stuporosed (complete physical immobility) Obstinate
Hebephrenic (undifferentiated)	Disharmony between mood and thought Social isolation Auditory hallucinations Bizarre delusions (hypochondriacal)
Residual (long-term)	Emotionally flattened Poor social skills Lack of initiative Internalised delusional system

Explanatory note: Isobel is suffering from a behavioural condition called *schizophrenia*. Although this is a general description of behaviour and that behaviour can vary from patient to patient, there are several main types.

Isobel's intense and irrational suspicion identifies her as paranoid. It is worth stating that one of the great problems faced by the nursing staff is that her suspicions are often confounded and reinforced by her having to take medication she doesn't think she needs, remaining in hospital against her wishes, and being questioned about her beliefs, which she already finds disturbing. It stands to reason that any care offered must be done skilfully and honestly. No attempt must be made to force her to do anything she does not want to, and where possible within the confines of her section, she should be permitted as much personal freedom as possible. The objective of the nurse must be to try and establish a trusting relationship with Isobel so that she can rely on one person at least,

A delusion is a false belief, often extremely bizarre, held with strength in the face of logical argument, which may conflict with the individual's sociocultural background, gender and environment

A hallucination is a false perception without an external stimulus, which can affect any of the five senses

thus reducing her ever present feelings associated with the threat to her personal safety.

The picture is also complicated by an active delusional system. If (as is probably the case with Isobel) these false beliefs are reinforced by hallucinations then it becomes extremely difficult for the nurse to orientate the patient to what is really happening. The secret is not to disagree, but not to agree with the patient either. The nurse must talk calmly and try to establish just what the individual wants to say, and always be honest and tell the truth. It will not help the individual if, simply for an easy life, the nurse agrees that someone from Mars is coming to broadcast her thoughts to the nation.

Delusions and their effects

Delusional type	Response
Persecutory	Highly suspicious of everyone Convinced people are out to do him harm
Jealousy	Others are extremely jealous of him Convinced people are against him because they envy him
Grandiose	Believes he is someone or something of great splendour. Often this is used as a reason for why people wish to harm him (as he is important)
Reference	Trifling, insignificant details both in conversation and environment have particular significance for him alone
Erotic	Others secretly admire him Convinced he is important because of the admiration he believes others have for him
Litigatious	People wish to do him harm through the legal system Convinced he has to employ lawyers to defend him in court

FIRST WEEK

Isobel progressively worsened in the next few days. Her thought disorder became more marked until all her sentences were based on a loose association of words and meanings. She was even more convinced that she was the subject of an evil plot and refused her medication regularly. On more than one occasion, she was violent towards the nursing staff, and she refused to be visited by her husband. In her favour she never tried to leave the ward, never threatened other patients, improved her personal hygiene and presentation, and seemed to enjoy keeping her room in good order. Several times she had to receive her medication by intramuscular injection. Her chlorpromazine had been increased to 200mg four times daily and because she began to exhibit stiffness of the joints and some difficulty in articulating her words, she was given Disipal (orphenadrine) 50mg four times daily to counteract these Parkinsonian type side effects.

NURSING CARE

Assessment

Whenever possible, Isobel would cut herself off from everyone around her, and it became increasingly difficult to communicate with her for any length of time. The following assessment of her unmet needs was made.

Physical
1 Poor sleep pattern, as little as three hours some nights.
2 No real physical exercise.
3 Eats very little, only picking at her meals, and seldom enjoying her food.
4 Poor eliminatory pattern.
5 Personal hygiene varied, but she had begun bathing each day.

Psychological
1 She remained frightened, suspicious and felt unsafe.
2 She found it difficult to distinguish between reality, and what was going on inside her own head. Delusions and hallucinations were real for Isobel, which made them even more alarming when she expressed them.

3 She had no insight into the true nature of her behaviour.
4 Her self image was extremely poor with a mistaken perception of her role.

Sociological

1 No real contact with other patients and only limited interaction with staff.
2 Refused to see members of her family.
3 She was very lonely.

The nursing team had already established their priorities in Isobel's case as the week progressed, and the assessment data only confirmed their decisions.

1 Isobel does not feel safe in any environment because of her belief that she is being threatened by an unnamed agency.
2 Because of her misinterpretation of events she has become isolated from other people, and now is unable to trust.

NURSING CARE

Objectives

The nursing diagnoses were discussed with Isobel and to a certain extent she agreed with them, although she did seem agitated when they were mentioned. It is important that the objectives set for her are understood by her, and that she can achieve them with reasonable ease. Her initial objectives from her first day's hospitalisation had not been achieved fully in that she had been unable to get along with her primary nurse, and had become verbally aggressive on occasions. These objectives needed refinement, and ought to be more clearly described to her so that she knew what was expected of her.

1 Will not avoid the primary nurse when she is approached by her.
2 Will discuss feelings of isolation and loneliness.

Delusional and perceptional activities are false beliefs, ideas and hallucinations experienced by the individual which interfere with his ability to understand what is really happening

In other words, Isobel was being asked to look more carefully at those things she knew to be real, her feelings, and not pay quite so much attention to those areas of her behaviour which others could not experience, i.e. her delusional and perceptional activities.

Explanatory note: it is important for patients, such as Isobel, to fully understand what is happening to them. It is wrong to assume that, if left alone, their behaviour will simply change for the better. Being disturbed, distressed, lonely and frightened by everything around you does not become more tolerable in isolation. The nurse's greatest asset is her ability to help orientate the patient with what is going on around her, and distract her from the unreal thoughts, beliefs and perceptions that torment her. The nurse must try to help the patient gain an appreciation of her own behaviour and through carefully constructed objectives guide her to some degree of insight and inner safety. The nurse can only hope to achieve this if the patient is involved as much as possible in this care activity. The nurse must never assume that a patient is too unwell to be involved, or too disturbed to understand. The patient's behaviour may well become more disturbed because the nurse fails to attempt the above.

| NURSING CARE |

Intervention

It was important to maintain constant communication between all team members, and Isobel's family was included in this. The increase in trust requisite for Isobel to regain her self image and composure would only come about through the growth of relationships, and in particular, those with her nurses. They must be as flexible and optimistic in her presence, being open and honest with her. Their use of empathy, i.e. trying to see how Isobel felt about what was happening to her, and being able to discuss it with her, was their main objective. She needed help to understand her own feelings, to come to terms with them and to establish some pattern for the future. In their interactions with her the nurses could not afford the luxury of making value judgements about what she said and did, nor could they criticise her behaviour in any way. They had to show that they accepted her as she was, and that they only wanted to help her overcome her feelings of fear and loneliness, in effect helping her achieve what she really wanted. They should respect her right to privacy; even in Isobel's case, a little solitude had to be allowed. If they spent all their time encouraging Isobel to talk, following her around and asking her to participate, she would become frustrated at the lack of personal time available to her. It was vital to find a happy medium between the needs of care, i.e. reality orientation, and the needs of the individual in personal choice.

The nursing team attempted to achieve these care objectives, using the following techniques:

1 Exaggerate trust activities and principles.
2 Always be accessible and approach Isobel whenever possible.
3 Ensure wherever possible that they did not require anything of Isobel when approaching her. If she spoke to nurses only when she had to take medication, eat, sleep, wash, or discuss objectives, she would suspect their motives towards her.
4 Respect her personal space.
5 Always listen to what she had to say.
6 Develop mutually agreeable objectives.
7 Discuss her feelings and try to identify in what ways they affected her behaviour.
8 Always keep calm in her presence.
9 Provide a restful environment for her, not pushing her into occupational areas if she did not wish to go there.
10 Maintain confidentiality, but make certain that she was aware that each nurse was part of the team.

11 Restrict contact to primary team only so that she would be able to identify them more easily. In this way, she might develop ties to one or two nurses rather than feel she had to share her innermost emotions and thoughts with a large group of people, some of whom she might not care to trust.

12 Monitor the effects of her medication.

13 Encourage her interest in personal hygiene, assisting her if necessary.

14 Encourage exercise, especially outside the ward, accompanied by a nurse.

15 Involve her family in her care and encourage them to visit as often as possible. Isobel must see that her family cared about her even though her circumstances were unfortunate at the present time. The family has to feel that they are doing something useful otherwise their feelings might develop into resentment towards Isobel. This type of family therapy forms the basis of Isobel's after care once she has been rehabilitated and left the confines of the psychiatric ward.

Explanatory note: it is all too easy for nursing staff to forget that the close relatives of patients in hospital have their own set of problems to contend with. Excluding them from the patient's care activities only tends to increase their feelings of isolation and frustration. When patients are suffering some form of psychiatric response, the relatives' difficulties are often exacerbated because the behaviour of their loved one is so unusual, frightening and often hurtful.

It is important for both the patient and the relatives that they have some part to play in the care proceedings. This can initially take the form of simple rotational visits, that is, members of the family visiting on their own as often as possible to ensure that a long period of contact is maintained with the patient. If all the family members visit at the same time, the visit may be over in one hour; if they visit individually the patient has company for three to four hours. Thus the patient retains contact with those people with whom she is most comfortable and the relatives gain an insight into the care

Psychiatric response means responding to everyday life situations in totally inappropriate ways giving rise to some form of psychiatric behaviour

activities provided. Also, if each family member has a set time to visit, a pattern develops and visiting appears less haphazard.

The nursing staff must spend time with the family, exploring ways of coping with the patient's behaviour and explaining its possible causes. In this way the relatives gain some understanding of the dynamics of the condition, and some of the mystery is lost.

The final stage is actually involving the relatives in treatment sessions, care evaluations and planning meetings which, of course, should also include the patient. The relatives should be encouraged to make observations about the effectiveness of what is happening to the patient and their own part in it. In other words the nurse should try to make the relatives feel part of the care team and not just unwanted observers. Eventually such involvement will prepare both patients and their relatives for the return home as neither will have lost contact with the other and each will know what to expect of the other.

NURSING CARE

Isobel
Response to interventions
Degree of insight
Recognition of personal difficulties
Amount of residual delusional ideas remaining
Identification of accurate life role
The desire to change her approach to her life role
The willingness to participate in her own recovery

Evaluation

Isobel spent almost four months on the psychiatric ward. The anti-psychotic medication helped to combat the delusional and perceptional disturbances she had, and in part, the intervention of the nursing staff assisted her to develop some limited insight into her feelings and behaviour. When her section expired after 28 days, she remained in hospital as an informal patient; if she had still resisted treatment at that time, it might have been necessary to transfer her to a treatment section (3), so that her programme could continue. However, with the continued support of her family and the re-introduction of her fortnightly injections of Modecate (fluphenazine decanoate) 25mg, she was able to return to her own home. She was not totally recovered, but with visits from her community psychiatric nurse, and careful monitoring of her behaviour, it was hoped that her progress would be enhanced by a return to a more normal life setting. She left

Nursing
Quality of nursing input
Method of delivery
Suitability of intervention
Frequency of evaluations
Individual nurse evaluations

hospital with a greater knowledge of her own feelings, a more positive approach to her ideas about her role within the family, and some insight into the behaviour she had used to avoid coming to terms with her family role. She and her family were encouraged to join the local branch of the Schizophrenic Society, a mutual self help group designed for the sufferers and families of Isobel's type of behaviour. She also returned regularly to the hospital to participate in the social activities of the ex-patient group.

TEST YOURSELF

1 List as many of the behavioural problems that Isobel presented as possible.

2 Why, in cases such as Isobel's, is it possible for the individual to become distressed, frightened, and at times aggressive?

3 Outline the main objectives of care for a patient who is suffering from a psychotic response to stress.

4 Describe, using the text, the methods used by the nursing team to develop a trusting relationship with someone who is highly suspicious of their motives.

FURTHER READING

MILES, P. 1984. Schizophrenia: An inside story. *New Society*, **68**, 14 June: 439–40.
SILVANO, A. 1979. *Understanding and Helping the Schizophrenic*. New York: Basic Books.
WARD, M. F. 1984. The nursing process in acute psychiatry, in *The Nursing Process in Psychiatry*: 149–67. Edinburgh: Churchill Livingstone.

8 Tony, who is highly over-active

HISTORY

Tony, a 28-year-old self employed builder, had been under a considerable amount of personal pressure recently. His order books were well filled, and in the evenings he was completing the final touches to his own self built house into which he and his wife hoped to move soon. Unfortunately, things had not gone quite as well as Tony had planned them, and the strain of having to pursue virtually two separate jobs simultaneously began to show.

At first, Tony became rather boisterous, shouting a great deal and generally appearing to be 'on top of the world'. However, his sleep pattern changed until in one week he had less than 25 hours sleep. He began to lose weight and wouldn't eat because he did not have the time for it. His degree of over-activity became more obvious. The men who worked for him found his excited behaviour difficult to handle and one of them did not turn up for work half-way through the week. This left Tony with even greater stress. By the weekend, he was 'feeling marvellous', but was worrying everyone else. Work on his own house had virtually stopped as he could not concentrate on any one project for more than a few minutes. His degree of over-activity meant that he would not sleep at all and he began calling customers, or potential customers, in the middle of the night to discuss business propositions. Needless to say, his wife was distressed by the whole affair. She had been kept awake during Tony's outbursts of over-activity and was beginning to feel the effects of lack of sleep. Her tolerance of Tony diminished and they began to argue with Tony always taking the upper hand. Eventually she went to see her G.P. because Tony refused to go himself, stating that he had far too much work to do. In effect, his usefulness, as both a boss and a worker, had ceased, because despite his apparently endless vitality, his judgement was poor, his decision making ability hampered by his lack of insight and hastiness, and his concentration span was extremely limited.

Factors influencing Tony's overactivity

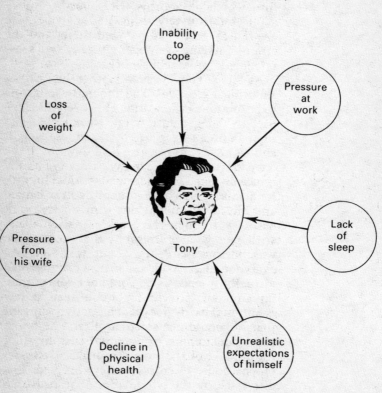

His G.P. agreed to visit Tony on site and although it was an unusual consultation, with Tony demonstrating his ability to carry several very heavy concrete blocks on his head, it was very easy to see that he was unwell and required hospitalisation. Quite apart from his psychological state, physically he was overtired, losing weight rapidly, and very dehydrated. Psychologically he was unable to rest although he considered himself perfectly fit and healthy. Moreover, he felt that he was able to carry out feats of amazing strength and endurance and thus was becoming something of a threat to himself. Socially, he had caused considerable difficulties between himself and his friends and relatives, and people began to treat him as a source of amusement.

Tony agreed to admission simply because he wanted to prove that there was nothing wrong with him. Once he arrived on the ward, he said he would demonstrate to all concerned just how fit he was.

ADMISSION TO THE WARD

Tony, accompanied by his wife and G.P., arrived on the ward and immediately plunged the whole place into confusion. He began jumping, cartwheeling and somersaulting all around the day area, betting people that he could manage all sorts of acrobatics. Attempts to calm him down were met with little success and he continued this way for several minutes. The nursing staff decided not to reinforce this behaviour and observed him from a distance, quite unobtrusively. Nobody laughed, or goaded Tony, and eventually he became bored with what he was doing, not to mention rather worn out. The remainder of his admission was reasonably quiet while he recovered his energy. However, he was easily stimulated, with a poor concentration span, and even simple word associations left him talking in circles. He had grandiose thoughts about his own abilities and was intolerant of criticism.

Instead of admitting Tony in the usual way, the primary nurse elected to do so in a quiet, slightly darkened room away from the main area. In this way it was hoped to reduce the amount of stimulus he received, and create an environment which in itself would induce a restful state. To a degree this strategy was successful in that he remained in the room and his physical activities were greatly subdued.

The psychiatrist's interview with Tony was equally as difficult as the initial nursing interview. Thus, the team decided that their immediate priority for care had to be to slow Tony down in some way, so that both his mind and his body would have an opportunity to rest. He was prescribed Largactil (chlorpromazine) 200mg three times daily, with the possibility of a further 200mg at night, if required. Because of the high dosage, he was also prescribed Disipal (orphenadrine) 50mg three times daily to counter probable extrapyramidal tract side effects from the major tranquilliser. The nursing staff were to monitor the effects of this medication while trying to provide a stimulus reduced environment in which he could function. The major concern of the nursing team, at this time, was that Tony might simply wear himself out and develop physical symptoms that would endanger his life.

The extra-pyramidal tract is the nerve pathways coming from the brain responsible for the maintenance of muscle tone

Stimuli reduced environment means nursing an individual in a quiet, darkened room and controlling the amount of sensory stimuli they receive. This has a calming effect upon the overactive

Explanatory note: the overactive patient, or manic patient, traditionally faced the possibility of total exhaustion and possible death. Dehydration, lack of nourishment and of sleep tended to self destruction. Without proper medical and nursing intervention, it was impossible for him to control his activities; because it was impossible for those caring for him to keep up with his outrageous behaviour, he was often left to his own devices. In the 1950s, with the advent of the Phenothiazine group of drugs, it became possible to give medication that would slow the individual down, control some of his psychotic behaviour, and yet not put him to sleep. Being able to nurse a patient whose level of consciousness had not been reduced meant that a more insight directed approach could be adopted. In Tony's case the nursing team had the chance to offer both a restful environment and personal contact at the same time. They were also able to construct a profile of him so that the intervention provided after his initial days of hospitalisation could be directed at his individual response to his behaviour and stress rather than provide blanket care for 'the manic patient'.

Initial stages

Tony was nursed in a quiet, darkened side room by the same nursing personnel each day. They produced a rota so that they did not have to spend a large amount of time with him because his behaviour was tiring to the staff. Their responses to his actions became more difficult to keep calm. They maintained his fluid balance chart and provided large amounts of fluids for him to drink.

Small snacks, sandwiches, crackers, etc. were left in his room for him to eat whenever he felt like it, but he was not expected to follow any particular routine, nor forced to indulge in protracted activities. It was hoped that, despite his short attention span and grandiose ideas, he might be prompted to combat his physical discrepancies. The nurses decided to talk little but to listen intently to what he had to say, not to provoke him into demonstrating his physical prowess and to manipulate his restlessness to divert his attention away from potential harmful activities. No attempt was made at this point to discuss his reason for admission and those things which might have precipitated his behavioural change.

Insight directed means activities designed to help the individual understand what is happening to him and why

| NURSING CARE |

Nursing response
Encourage him to drink as much fluid as possible
Maintain his sleep and fluid balance charts
Limit staff involved with him to a minimum and organise a rota system
Talk quietly to him
Nurse in a quiet darkened room
Reduce stimulus as much as possible
Listen to what he has to say without over-responding
Monitor weight
Keep him supplied with small snacks
Promote rest and encourage sleep
Reduce stimuli at night and create a good environment in which to sleep
Use diversional techniques when his behaviour becomes too excessive

Observations

Much of the profile data for Tony was gained
from talking to his wife. She said that he was a
man whose mood was often difficult to predict. For a time he would be happy and cheerful
with plenty of life, and then for no apparent
reason he would become sullen and morose
and find little to occupy himself (cyclothymic
personality). He had been this way for as long
as she had known him and was indeed very
much like his father who, it was discovered,
had a long history of admissions to psychiatric
units for manic depressive illness. Tony himself had never been admitted, but on several
occasions in the past, his wife had been worried about his behaviour. His moments of
crisis usually coincided with periods of high
stress and acute changes in routine. At one
stage, he suspected his wife of infidelity, and in
another, he had been taken to court because he
had failed to honour a contract with a client.
He was generally a generous and cheerful man
who worked hard and was ambitious.

The observations made from Tony's actual
behaviour on the ward showed that his
fluctuations in mood had swung very much in
the direction of over-activity, or mania.

A cyclothymic personality is a type of personality, quite normal, where the individual tends to have obvious 'ups and downs' in his level of mood

Physical

1 Dry mouth, constantly sweating, dehydrated.
2 Constipated – no bowel action since
  admission.
3 Pulse and B/P quite high, no real recovery
  following attempts at physical exertion.
4 Poor food intake. Only eats snacks, milk
  drinks, etc. Has no time to sit and eat at
  table.
5 Maximum of four hours of sleep per night,
  although he is more restful now than on
  admission.

6 Restless and physically over-active whenever the opportunity arises or his concentration wavers.

7 Poor attention to personal hygiene. Will not bathe and washing is minimal.

Psychological

1 Mentally over-active resulting in flights of ideas, disjointed speech, loose association phrases. These racing thoughts make conversation and concentration difficult for him.

2 Poor judgement. Decisions made by him are often totally without forethought and reflect no estimation of the consequences of his actions.

3 Poor concentration span, often as little as 2 or 3 seconds.

4 Excited and uncontrollable at times; his mood fluctuates from being merely very happy to being boisterous.

5 Easily distracted – because of poor concentration.

6 Often becomes easily bored, then irritable.

7 Rather intolerant of criticism – argues with people who do not agree with everything he says.

8 Has grandiose ideations about his own abilities, from simply saying he can drink more milk and drink it faster than any man alive (and trying to prove it), to insisting he can fly and, unless distracted, attempting to prove that also! This inflated view of his self image and self esteem creates difficulties which go far beyond the confines of his own environment. He has on several occasions made telephone calls promising work and money to people which are totally unrealistic for him at present.

Sociological

1 Impossible to hold any real conversation with him because of his grandiosity and poor concentration.

Loose association phrases are a speech pattern characterised by statements of little relationship linked only by similar sounding words or a wandering train of thought

Ideation is a group of thoughts and feelings as a consequence of an original idea

2 Has been unable to make any positive steps towards interactions or relationships with other patients on the ward. This is partially due to being limited to his own room for most of the time. Even when he is moving around, however, he is only demonstrating his own capabilities. He is very egotistical in his approach to anyone or anything.

3 Has frightened several of the other patients with his physical antics.

4 He is over extravagant towards others and, because he fails to live up to his promises, is seen as a figure of ridicule by some.

5 Has no real social conscience, having dropped his trousers in the day room on more than one occasion.

Tony was seen, therefore, as a disinhibited over-active individual with no insight into his unacceptable behaviour. The degree of mental over-activity he was experiencing was the influencing factor in his presentation because it meant he was unable to consider in any detail the daily running of his own life. Probably more seriously he also could not sort out the perceptional information he received from his environment for the purpose of making accurate decisions. He was, in short, a liability to himself and a very difficult patient to nurse objectively. Much of what the nursing team was doing at this time involved simply trying to stop him from becoming even more stimulated and excited.

Perceptional information is received by the special senses about one's external and internal environment

NURSING CARE

Assessment

After a period of several days, the whole of Tony's situation was assessed with a view to constructing a realistic programme of care that was not simply designed to inhibit his activities but more to help him come to terms with his feelings and to do something constructive about his own behaviour. The main areas of concern were still his physical over-activity which resulted in weight loss, dehydration and poor eliminatory functions. Most of this, of course, was due to his mental activities but the effects of restricted environment, low stimulation regimes and the anti-psychotic medication were already beginning to be felt.

NURSING CARE

Evaluation

It was also important at this stage to evaluate the effectiveness of the initial nursing intervention for Tony. The primary team, and in some cases, those nurses who had been used to augment the team, discussed Tony's response to them while being nursed in the rather restricted environment they had selected for him. Generally speaking they found him a difficult person to nurse, mainly because he required constant supervision, and his nurse needed to be aware of her effect upon him with every action or statement she made. They considered several of the interventions in relation to his over-activity and others in relation to his physical well being. It was generally agreed that their care had been appropriate to the situation, and in line with their assessment of his current mental state, would form a good basis upon which he could begin to regain his recovery.

1 Over-active due to his inability to come to terms with his own responsibilities.
2 Poor fluid intake, unless prompted, resulting in dehydration.

These two areas, though by no means covering every eventuality in Tony's presentation, were considered those that held the key to his recovery.

Evaluation of initial nursing intervention designed to
reduce Tony's mental activity

Intervention	Evaluation
Quiet darkened environment to reduce stimuli	Achieved
Regular rota of familiar faces to reduce stimuli	Achieved
Not responding to constant talking	Achieved
Distracting him when he is overactive	Achieved
Changing staff regularly so that they are always fresh and spontaneous	Not always achieved

Evaluation of initial nursing intervention designed to
promote an increase in Tony's well being

Intervention	Evaluation
Provision of small snacks at any time of day	Achieved
Weight gain	Achieved
Some concentration of personal hygiene activities (confined to his room)	Achieved
Constant provision of fluids	Achieved
Mouth care for effects of dehydration on teeth, gums, lips	Achieved
Provision of quiet darkened environment in the evening to promote sleep response	Not always achieved

NURSING CARE

Objectives

The objectives have to reflect not only the need to provide a more relaxing approach to daily life and the adequate re-hydration necessary to return Tony's body to a more optimal physical level, but they also have to be functional, providing him with realistic and potentially rewarding achievements. They must be positive and centre around those areas of his behaviour that provide him with the most satisfaction. The key, of course, was still to slow him down and provide rest, so the first objective has this as its basis.

1 Tony will identify for himself a realistic programme of daily activities that will include periods of rest. He will try to stick to this regime.

2   Tony is to continue to remain in the company of his nursing team member during scheduled discussion times, even though he might wish to do something else.
3   To gain a more enlightened view of his situation, he should discuss with the primary nurse the recent events in his life which might have caused his distress and discomfort.

The final objective was quite simply:

4   Tony will drink 200ml of fluid each hour.

As this change in emphasis of care was initiated, so too was Tony's involvement in it. He was actually encouraged to help in the construction of the care objectives which enabled the nursing team the opportunity to broaden the conversation to include his behaviour, responsibilities and thoughts on hospitalisation.

The third objective was extremely important because, hopefully, Tony would be in a position to identify precipitants in his recent past. When considered more closely under the guidance of the nursing team, these precipitants would give him a clearer picture of what was happening to him. Also if in doing so he was able to reflect on his feelings towards those events, rather than shrouding them in mental over-activity, he might be in a better position to cope with their recurrence in a more acceptable fashion.

Explanatory note: the conditions of mania and depression are closely linked. Many argue that they are, in fact, different presentations of the same illness and that both are manifestations of psychotic depression. It is not uncommon to see excessively happy and boisterous individuals, such as Tony, suddenly and for no apparent reason burst into tears and be inconsolable for long periods of time. It is difficult to say accurately whether this is caused by a true depression or is simply a response to the mental confusion that is created by the lack of concentration and flights of ideas. The nurse, however, must be aware that beneath the façade of 'super happiness', the individual is very often unhappy. The two presentations, when rather better controlled by either anti-depressants on the one hand or major tranquillisers on the other, are usually treated with the same drug – Lithium Carbonate – which controls the mood of both groups of individuals. A clearer picture of why this should be can be gained by considering the pre-morbid personality of the individual which, in Tony's case, was inclined towards a raising or lowering of mood in this rather obvious way. We all have our bad and good days, but in Tony's case this was much more marked. When there is an increase in pressure or stress, it will have the effect of accentuating whatever current mood he is in.

Depressive and manic reactions to stress

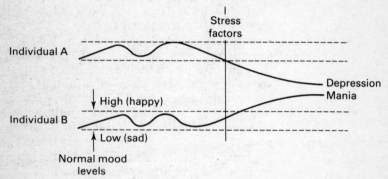

NURSING CARE

Intervention

The nursing intervention for Tony was designed to:

increase his commitment to his own physical well being;

decrease his over-activeness;

increase his knowledge of why he was behaving as he was;

give him the opportunity to make accurate decisions about his future, so that he could avoid such a situation recurring, or at least recognise the initial signs and do something about it before he had to be readmitted, and consequently inhibit his life style.

1. The production of small meals, regular fluids, etc. to maintain his progress in physical recovery.
2. Maintain fluid balance charts and keep regular checks on TPR and BP.
3. Try not to restrict his movements, but offer alternatives when he starts to become hyper-active, i.e. constructive, creative activities.
4. Use diversional tactics whenever his conversation becomes stylised and repetitive. Help him to overcome his racing thoughts by forcing him to concentrate on his feelings and responses to what is going on around him. Encourage rest periods, and help him to sleep by supplying warm drinks and quietened environment. Listen to what he is saying at such times but do not stimulate him into further conversation by talking unnecessarily.
5. Do not encourage outrageous behaviour.
6. Do not laugh at his antics.
7. Maintain a safe environment for him, and divert him from potentially hazardous activities and areas.
8. Encourage discussion about his list of ideas leading up to his admission.
9. Discuss his feelings towards these events.
10. Initially accompany his wife during visits so that she is not over-taxed by his behaviour and acts negatively towards him. Talk to her about the objectives of his care and involve her in the therapeutic elements of his conversational programme.
11. Monitor effects of medication.
12. Try to establish a rapport with him that enhances the patient/nurse relationship and, in particular, elements of trust, acceptance and caring.

Rehabilitation

Tony responded well to the care he was offered and gradually became more involved in the production and methods of applying the interventions. As he developed more control over his behaviour, in line with a reduction in his mental over-activity, he was able to counter the more bizarre elements of his grandiose ideas and racing thoughts. To a degree the nurses were able to restrict his grandiosity by never challenging his statements or asking for proof of his prowess.

By not denying his image of himself, there was less need for Tony to demonstrate his talents; on the occasions when he did, his behaviour was not reinforced by laughter or adulation, and it became a less profitable method of acting. His main source of behavioural reinforcement came from being able to do the things he wanted to do, an increase in his personal space and involvement in creative activities – for all of which he received praise, from his wife and the nursing team. In all, he remained on the ward for two months. During that time he was transferred from Largactil to Lithium Carbonate to control his mood swings. The effects were rewarding, but it would be necessary for him to continue taking the medication for many years.

Personal space is a term used to describe an individual's personal choices and the ability to be free to carry them through or experience them

Evaluation

Tony had to consider several points which might have a bearing on his ability to maintain an independent and worthwhile life style on his return to the community.

1   How had his decision making ability been affected?
2   Had his social skills been impaired in any way?

3 How did he perceive his personal relationships?

4 How did he see his own personal identity?

5 What was his commitment to work?

6 What were his intentions for the future?

7 Could he recognise the feelings he experienced which eventually led to his becoming over-active, and if so, how might he be able to use that knowledge to counteract any further episode?

<table>
<tr><td>

TEST YOURSELF

</td><td>

1 Identify the kind of person who might be predisposed to becoming excessively over-active as a response to stress.

2 What were the major physical/psychological/sociological factors in Tony's presentation?

3 Outline three important areas of concern for the nursing team when constructing Tony's care plan.

4 Describe a programme of intensive nursing intervention to help the over-active individual regain self control and a more realistic approach to daily living.

</td></tr>
</table>

FURTHER READING

BUCKWALTER, K. C. & KERFOOT, K. M. 1982. Emergency department nursing care of the manic patient. *Journal of Emergency Nursing*, **8**, 5: 239–42.

IRONBAR, N. O. 1983. Mania – Unit 4 in Self instruction in *Psychiatric Nursing*. London: Baillière Tindall.

MCDERMOTT, J. 1983. Ready or not, here comes the patient on Lithium. *Nursing* (U.S.), **13**, 8: 234–6.

9 George, who has been in hospital for many years

Introduction

For most people in a psychiatric ward, admission means relief from the ever present stress of symptoms, the opportunity to assess how those symptoms affect their ability to function as an independent individual, and the chance under professional guidance to plan a realistic and hopeful future. For some people, however, re-admission at some future date and the inevitability of a long stay in hospital are a more realistic outlook.

Psychiatric patients, because of the nature of their condition and their response to it, are prone to this situation more than any other, though factors such as personality, motivation, duration of illness and the care provided are all likely to influence what happens to them. In time, constant exposure to the limitations of hospital life produce lethargy, a lack of insight into their plight, lack of self interest, lack of social skills, no motivation for change and adaptability, all of which inhibit their chances of recapturing their original place in society. The possibility of rehabilitation which should, in effect, begin on admission, will be further influenced by facilities available in the community for support purposes, the involvement of family and friends, and the attitudes of the society to which they are returning. In short, the longer they remain in hospital cut off from the real word, the more difficult it becomes to actually get them back into society.

Factors influencing the pace of an individual's discharge

Hospital factors	Community factors	Personal factors
Length of stay in hospital	Community resources	Severity of condition
Hospital rehabilitation policy	Support of family/friends	Type of behaviour used
Medication	Accommodation/finance/ work	Factors precipitating admission
Degree of institutionalisation	Stigma	Amount of behaviour remaining
	Attitude of community	Motivation
	Links with community	Personality
	Voluntary or self-help groups	Self-confidence
	Day care facilities	Feelings of rejection
	Case load of community team	Insight into behaviour

| HISTORY |

George, at 52 years of age, unmarried and with 9 years of hospitalisation behind him, is just such a man.

His aged parents live quite close to the hospital, but in recent years they have visited him less and less and he has not been to their house for over two years. He is very set in his ways, following daily rituals and routines imposed on him partly because of his illness and partly because of the institution itself. A return to the community for him would be a long and involved process which will never come to fruition if he cannot become actively involved in the motivational cycle necessary for him to want to leave hospital. He has little or no personal money, no real job prospects although he was employed in various jobs until he was 40 years old. If his parents are not prepared to have him live with them, either because they feel threatened by him or because of guilt or stigma, then he has no accommodation and no friends or social role to return to.

The motivational cycle: an awareness of the desire for something, produces behaviour designed to achieve it. In turn this generates an awareness of more needs

Despite receiving depot injections of Depixol (flupenthixol) 80mg fortnightly to alleviate his psychotic characteristics and his withdrawn and lethargic approach plus Kemadrin (procyclidine hydrochloride) 2.5mg three times daily (to counteract the extra pyramidal effects of the depixol), he still exhibits residual symptoms of his condition, especially when confronted with the possibility of change in his routines.

The staff on his ward, however, are concerned that the longer he remains in the enclosed environment of the hospital, the more futile his life will become, and his basic rights as an individual will be denied him because of his disability.

They started to carefully monitor his daily routine, and to establish exactly what his patterns of behaviour were in different situations and towards different people around the hospital. In this way they hoped to establish an overall picture of George's behavioural skills and his levels of adaptability.

Recreational areas
(Shop/social
club/cafeteria)

↕

Occupational area
(Workshops)

↕

Social events
(Ward based/inter-
ward/interhospital)

↕

In company of
visitors
(Personal or
official)

↕

Clinical area
(Ward
environment)

Explanatory note: when patients receiving continuous care leave the ward to go to other departments either for recreation, occupation or simply to get a cup of tea from the shop/canteen, they very often present a different picture from that which is regarded as being their 'normal' in the ward. The problem for the ward staff is that after continued exposure to their patients on the ward, they tend to see them only in that light. Despite the fact that they may visit patients in occupational therapy, accompany them on outings and mix with them during social occasions, etc. the type, mode and differences of behaviour adopted by the patients during those occasions may be seen as transitory and not part of the individual's alternatives. None of us behave the same each day, nor for that matter do we behave the same way to the same situation each time, but we do become identified with a certain type of behaviour. If we stray from it and behave slightly differently, we are still identical people and have not changed into someone else. However, people might ask you if something is wrong or simply accept that you are behaving differently. The long stay patient is just the same. He may be categorised as behaving in a certain way because that is his 'normal'.

However, when confronted with new situations or a more pleasant environment, or something which gives him pleasure he, just like everyone else, will vary his behaviour accordingly. It is important that these alterations in behaviour are recorded if the ward staff are to gain a true picture of the individual's capabilities, and in George's case, it is essential that the staff also note the stimuli that provoke the behavioural change.

NURSING CARE

Observations

It was agreed that the primary nurse would be responsible for collecting the data about George. She made it known to him what she was doing, anticipating some possible shift in his emotional level. No shifts were forthcoming, however, and he appeared to accept her outline of what she was doing without any real outward show of feeling. She must try to involve him in her observations, no matter how small his involvement, and she also had to ensure that he was aware of what was happening. If George felt something sinister was occurring, it was possible that he would react accordingly; she therefore should maintain a very high level of communication with him to overcome this potential problem.

She accompanied him around the hospital, not necessarily always at his side. She spoke to the people with whom he came into contact including therapy staff, ward staff, canteen staff and other patients. Wherever possible she tried talking to these people as soon after their meeting with George as possible in an attempt to reduce inaccurate observations.

During this period of time, she also gathered data about his activities in and around his own ward. To a certain extent much of this data would reinforce the existing profile of George's behaviour, but it was important to verify whether what was already accepted as being his 'normal' was indeed so.

Finally all the data gained from external and

internal sources was correlated, including a report obtained from the social worker about George's parents. Other information for consideration came from the occupational therapy staff who were already involved in a small skills programme with George.

Although much of the data gathered was of a negative nature, there were positive aspects of George's daily activities which needed to be noted separately. His eventual rehabilitation programme would actually centre upon enlarging this productive and rewarding behaviour.

They included:

Positive Observation

1 Getting himself dressed, feeding himself, keeping his own room reasonably tidy, regular toileting, good sleep pattern and being physically illness free – totally mobile if a little slow moving.

2 He saw himself as having dignity despite his hospitalisation. He had a role to play within the institution and the patient hierarchy. His psychological symptoms were reasonably well controlled, and did not limit his ability to function on a daily basis.

3 When visiting other areas around the hospital he was sociable towards those he met, recognising certain individuals and actually electing to spend time with them. Showed interest in recreational activities, though usually as a spectator. Particular interests included music and card games. He seemed to have two, possibly three special acquaintances in the hospital, all patients with whom he would spend considerable periods of time.

These observations showed that George had a social life, no matter how limited, which took up most of his day. As such he had an identity

Skills programme is therapy involving practice and reward to re-teach either social or life/living skills

and a purpose within the patient structure, and the primary nurse discovered that George was seen by other patients as being either 'a regular' or 'an important' patient.

Positive observational data about George

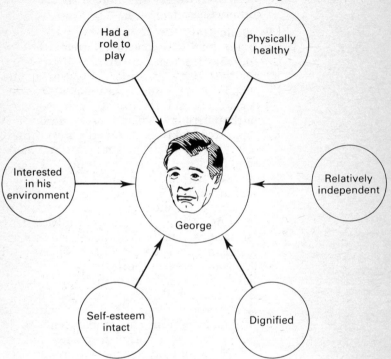

Interested in his environment → George

Had a role to play

Physically healthy

Relatively independent

Self-esteem intact

Dignified

Negative Observations
The negative observations indicate to the nursing team where they would most likely have to intervene if they were to increase George's quality of life, and subsequently the possibility of discharge.

Physical
1   Poor attention to personal hygiene and cleanliness of clothing. George would only bathe or wash when it was suggested to

him. Shaving was not a problem as he had grown a beard, but it looked rather scruffy.
2   Lack of exercise and volition. Not only did he rarely indulge in recreational activities but he had neither the desire nor the necessity to move around more than was absolutely essential.

Psychological

1   Emotionally he appeared flattened. He had no real fluctuations in his mood, being neither happy nor sad. This would only change when some variation in his routine occurred, and he might become angry, although that was never certain. In short he appeared ambivalent towards most things.
2   He showed little personal assertiveness, and his social skills were limited. He performed with little or no confidence in new or difficult circumstances, and always sought avoidance as the best method of dealing with potentially embarrassing situations. He tended to be submissive even in relationships with his peers, and showed no real authority.
3   His self image was incomplete and limited. He saw himself as being unimportant.
4   When asked about his current status, he had no insight into his problems nor could he see any real reason to change his life style. He did not consider himself to be disadvantaged in any way, yet he remained almost totally without stimulus.

Sociological

Many of the sociological difficulties were intermingled with the psychological ones, yet it was possible for the team to isolate particular social areas of concern:

1   Poor social competence. He really only mixed with three people and then in a very submissive fashion. He never took the initiative within these relationships and

when confronted with something he did not wish to do, he would simply opt out.

2 Used little verbal communication. His non-verbal communication, body posture, lack of eye contact, gestures and bearing, usually said, 'Leave me alone.'

Negative observational data about George

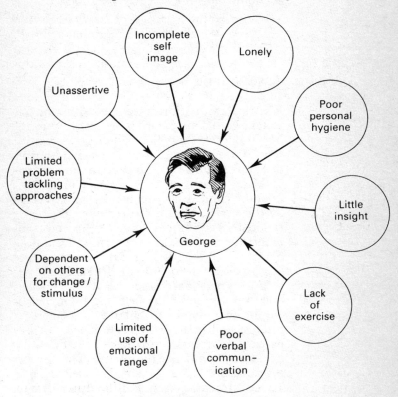

3 He placed the dependence for the running of his daily life upon others. He was never really prepared to tackle problems for himself and in fact appeared to have lost the facility for true problem solving.

4 There seemed to be a lowering of his personal standards in that he behaved in a

rather demeaning manner most of the time. He would regularly rummage through the ash trays to find cigarette ends, lounged about in the day area and used few of the social graces that he had once carried out without thought of doing so.

5 He seemed a lonely man, going nowhere, doing nothing. George's outlook on life was vague at best, heavily restricted at worst yet he never seemed maudlin or complaining.

NURSING CARE

Assessment

A critical evaluation of George's situation had to take into consideration his response to the hospital environment which, by nature, tended to be rather ritualistic and routine orientated. However, he gave the impression of being a man who was afraid of making mistakes, and as a consequence, being rejected by those around him. To remedy this, he restricted his activities as much as possible, thus reducing the risk of making errors. The initial objectives of the nursing team would have to be to pay attention to small details and increase his personal confidence. At a later stage, once his image of himself had improved, it would be possible to enlarge his sphere of interest. Ultimately he would need to pay particular attention to more specific skills necessary to enhance the quality of his life and his potential for personal independence. These, of course, would all be dependent on George's initial programme, and the degree of potential that he exhibited, so it was necessary to concentrate on the three immediate priorities of:

How to present himself to others
How to behave appropriately in given circumstances
How to communicate effectively
How to solve problems

1 Personal hygiene
2 Conversational skills
3 Simple problem tackling/solving

It was also imperative that George be involved in this increase in his care so that he would feel he had accomplished something. Even before the objectives were isolated, it was important to discuss the whole process with him without confusing him and without threatening his limited sense of security or altering his routines too much.

NURSING CARE

Intervention

The social worker's report indicated that George's parents were unwilling to have him home with them again because of their own age, routines and probable apprehension about his behaviour. George would require a considerable amount of care before he could be transferred to a hostel ward or discharged to unsupervised sheltered accommodation. Initially this care would centre around the three priority areas but it was important that it should be sufficiently stimulating and rewarding for him so that it might affect his overall presentation and performance.

For the problem of personal hygiene, he was asked about the possibility of washing and bathing on a regular basis. To remind him to do so would simply have meant that he was complying with staff wishes; it was necessary to discuss matters relating to cleanliness, washing, etc., and hope that he would make the decision for himself. His objective in this area was therefore:

> In one month's time, George will decide for himself to bathe a minimum of once a week and wash at least once each day.

To a degree this objective, and the method of care that went with it, were designed so that they created a problem solving situation for George. He would have to determine for him-

A hostel ward is a clinical area, often separate from the main hospital, run by the patients themselves with limited supervision from nursing staff. Its function is to prepare patients more realistically for discharge

self whether to wash or not, and what the consequences were for both sets of actions. His behaviour would be influenced by receiving a different form of conversation with the nursing team depending on his choice. His interests in recreational activities were used as the basis for conversation, and it soon became apparent that George enjoyed watching most sporting activities.

His major form of reward was playing a game of cribbage, at which he excelled. However, to heighten the motivation for problem solving, each week he was set simple problems, e.g. the cribbage board was hidden in different locations so that he had to find it. His objective was simply:

> Each week George will solve a simple task/problem outlined by the primary nurse which will become more difficult as his abilities increase.

Although the tasks themselves were simple, when considered from the point of view of someone regularly using realistic, positive solving techniques, for George they represented a considerable challenge. At first he would not be involved in the production of these problems, nor would he be aware that he was having to do anything out of the ordinary – he simply needed to stretch his imagination and increase his dynamic activities. At a later stage, he might well be included in the planning stage of the problems themselves, but not until he had regained some experience and confidence.

The area of conversational skills too had been covered by the reward system used to reinforce his bathing practice. However, it was not sufficient for him to simply respond to approaches, as this reflected his submissiveness; therefore, it was intended that he should

1 Will decide for himself to bathe once per week and wash once per day

Review in one month

2 Will solve one simple problem each week

Review in one month

3 Will greet his primary nurse before spoken to

Review in one month

Institutionalisation is a growing dependence by the individual upon the institution for the provision of all basic needs without the individual taking any responsibility for them himself

actually initiate some form of verbal interaction. His objective became:

> At the end of one month, George will greet his primary nurse before the nurse greets him.

It was necessary to talk to George at some length about this objective. In truth it was also important to ensure that he actually knew the name of the primary nurse because no one had ever heard him use the names of the staff on the ward, with the possible exception of when he spoke to the charge nurse.

Explanatory note: there are two points of interest here. Firstly, it is important for nurses to try and remember that due to the lack of social skills exhibited by many continuing care patients, they very often do not see the need to use names, or for that matter even remember them. Because of the nature of institutionalisation, the patient is unlikely to employ names because they represent companionship, belonging, friendship and commitment. Most of these elements are missing from the patient's current life style. The nurse must try to remember this when talking to such patients, introducing herself whenever possible, reminding them of her name at regular intervals and showing not only that it is all right for him to call her by name but that she actively encourages it.

Secondly, a large number of patients have lost many of their conversational skills, and more importantly they may have lost the ability to begin meaningful verbal interactions. An objective sequence must be constructed which will accurately reflect a gradual growth in the patient's capability and response to care. For example:

1 At the end of two weeks, 'the patient' will not move away from any member of staff who sits next to him.
2 At the end of two weeks, the patient will not move away from staff who sit next to him and will say 'good morning'.

And so on until at the end of two weeks, the patient will greet staff when they sit next to him. In George's case, of course, his level of competence did not require such a beginning but certainly his gradual progress would need to be carefully planned and executed.

Other members of the multi-disciplinary team were also involved in the care provided by the nursing team. The occupational therapy team reinforced the actions of the nurses while George was in their department, and likewise the nurses monitored the effects of the input of the occupational therapy staff. In view of his parents' reluctance to ever have him return to their home, his rehabilitation programme will have to include significant self support skills. The nurses will eventually have to help George cope with the possible rejection he might experience because of that fact.

Other items that would be incorporated into George's rehabilitation programme include:

1   The use of role play to act through situations before George encounters them in the outside world so that he gains confidence in his abilities, and is more prepared for the realism of social encounters.
2   Discussion of George's feelings so that he could give vent to his fears and hopes in a manner that might provide support and encouragement.
3   The allocation of simple tasks, linked to his problem solving objectives.
4   Educational, recreational and special interest visits out into the community, accompanied at first and later unsupervised.
5   Attendance at the social skills group.
6   Introduction to work practice, either in an industrial therapy unit, or around the hospital in a limited capacity.
7   Attempts to re-educate his parents about George's performance and potential including visits by him to his parents' home, initially accompanied by his primary nurse.
8   Discussion about his self image, social activities, and life expectation, with a view to enlarging his awareness of both himself and his environment.

9   Contact with local voluntary organisations
     at both social events and support groups.

It was essential that the nursing staff show
tolerance, a deep sense of personal interest,
and that they were prepared to take as much
time as was necessary.

NURSING
CARE

Evaluation

George's rehabilitation programme, if successful, will take several years to come to fruition,
but within the skills training programme,
several factors will dictate his degree of independence:

1   Punctuality, time keeping
2   Self control
3   Relationships with others, including re-
     settlement officer, social worker, etc.
4   Group participation
5   Assertiveness and social competence
6   Speech and eye contact
7   Listening and questioning ability
8   Paying attention and being quiet
9   Problem tackling approaches
10   Ability to cope with rejection and social
     stigma

The involvement of George in his own rehabilitation will remain the one constant
component of the evaluation. The nurses must
monitor the level of residual psychotic symptoms that he might present, in what circumstances and to what effect. More importantly,
they have to find a way of combating these
symptoms and continuing the rehabilitation
programme in spite of them.

Once the programme for George has been
initiated, it will be important to make regular
checks about the suitability of the care provided within it. It was only because of an

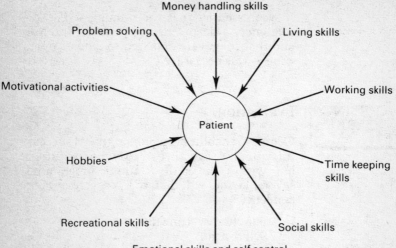

Final aims of a skills programme

Money handling skills

Problem solving

Living skills

Motivational activities

Working skills

Patient

Hobbies

Time keeping skills

Recreational skills

Social skills

Emotional skills and self control

evaluation of his care by the nurses that extra observational data were correlated. It would be of little value if the only reviews that took place coincided with care plan evaluations, as very often these evaluations only take place at four or five week intervals. Thus, at handovers or team meetings, a simple assessment of nursing performance would be necessary.

Other members of the multidisciplinary team should be made aware of the findings of these assessments as their input into the care programme may be influenced by the success or failure of individual interventions. Likewise reciprocal data from those other disciplines might influence the future strategies of the nurses. Two way communication channels are vital to the performance of all those involved in George's rehabilitation.

1 Outline the main presenting features of an individual who has been exposed to hospital life for a long period of time to include physical, psychological and sociological elements.

2 How do the loss of social skills inhibit the individual's ability to communicate effectively with others?

3 Describe a realistic approach by the nurse that would combat the immediate effects of institutionalisation.

FURTHER READING

STONE, K., PARKER, D., ABBOTT, K. & CHALKLEY, J. 1984. Making decisions. *Nursing Mirror*, **158**, 4 Jan, Mental Health Forum: ii–v.
WARD, M. F. 1985. The nursing process in continuing care psychiatry, in *The Nursing Process in Psychiatry*: 168–80. Edinburgh: Churchill Livingstone.
WILLARD, C. 1984. The story of John. *Nursing Mirror*, **158**, 4 Jan, Mental Health Forum: vii–viii.

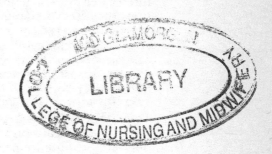

10 Constance, an elderly lady

Introduction

Far many more people today lead longer and healthier lives than ever before. This trend can be attributed to many factors, and not least of them would be the increase in medical technology, care facilities and nursing resources. For most of these people, retirement means a perfectly normal process of growing old with just as much excitement, sadness, success and failure as at any other stage in their lives. Yet for some, approximately one in ten in the UK, this continuous chain of events is prematurely interrupted by an organically orientated condition that affects their memory, general mental functioning and social involvement. This process of abnormal ageing, usually termed senile dementia, alters the whole pattern of the individual's senescence because they gradually lose contact both psychologically and sociologically with what is going on around them. Their lack of judgement, reduced personal safety, and susceptibility to physical deterioration often require tremendous support in the home from caring relatives. Unfortunately, for most sufferers the opportunity to remain either in their own home or in that of relatives becomes an impossibility because of the strain upon these carers. Hospital admission, initially for short periods of assessment, but later for more continuous care, becomes an inevitability.

Organically orientated condition is an illness caused because of physical changes in the body

Senile dementia: the term *chronic brain failure* is often used to describe this condition

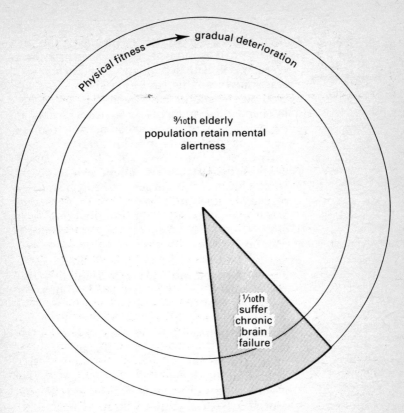

Incidence of chronic brain failure in the UK

In many respects, the admission of an ageing person to a psychiatric ward increases their disorientation because of the lack of familiarity with the new environment. The inability to memorise this new information and the potentially threatening presence of unrecognisable people, only heightens the difficulties. Add to this the possible sense of loss and guilt experienced by relatives, and it can be seen that such admissions need to be carried out with careful attention to detail and with a great deal of sensitivity.

HISTORY

Constance had been in hospital for nearly a year. At 71 years old she had no close relatives, and up until 18 months ago had been living in a warden controlled flat with her husband. It was known at this time that she was not as well as she might have been, and when her husband died suddenly of a heart attack, it became apparent that she had been extremely dependent on him for meeting nearly all of her daily needs. Only days after her husband's death, she set the kitchen alight by leaving the cooker on after she had gone to bed. She readily agreed to come into hospital, but then resisted the actual admission until the final moment, after a great deal of encouragement from the warden.

ADMISSION TO THE WARD

On admission, she had been frightened and apprehensive, and the nurse tried to show respect and sympathy for her by taking time to explain everything simply and quietly. Constance responded well to the nurse who listened carefully to what she said, and was patient and tolerant with her. Basically her admission had been solely for the purpose of assessing her capabilities to lead an independent life with a view to discharging her to some form of nursing home at a later date. Unfortunately, her condition deteriorated quite quickly in the first few weeks following admission until she had become isolated, withdrawn, sad and disorientated to a point that made her highly dependent on nursing intervention.

Explanatory note: as we grow older, we become dependent upon routines, practices and rituals which help us through our daily lives. They provide signposts that we can follow to give us confidence and self esteem. Above all else, they provide a sense of purpose and stimulation, but when measured against the faster pace of earlier life seem to have little real significance for the younger observer. At times they are regarded as eccentricities by the unimaginative, and seem to be worthless and irritating. More dangerously, they can be viewed as maladaptive or abnormal. The nurse must attempt to see the older patient as having a unique life style different to her own and accept the differences in approaches to living. Such things as sleep reversal, (sleeping during the day and staying awake at night), reminiscing and suspicion of change are common amongst the elderly, yet are often regarded as unnatural by a younger population who has yet to experience them. The need to understand the patient as having perhaps a different set of values, morals, beliefs and desires must be paramount in the nurse's approach if she is to care in an individualised way. Respect for the patient's memories and experience and a willingness to explore them together can often provoke a depth of insight on the part of the nurse that no amount of classroom tuition could ever produce.

Constance developed urinary incontinence, was found to be anaemic, and became disinterested in personal hygiene, eating and drinking. She was increasingly suspicious of the nurses and began hoarding relatively unconnected and apparently insignificant pieces of paper in her handbag. Her speech was limited to monosyllabic, monotoned responses and her interaction with others was nil. Even more disturbing for the nursing team was the information from the warden that it was suspected Constance had made a rather crude attempt at suicide about two years before but the whole affair had been covered up and forgotten. There was no previous history of psychiatric illness and thus it was assumed that Constance may have experienced great emotional trauma in coming to terms with her failing abilities and an awareness of her growing dependence upon her husband.

Constance remained in hospital because she simply did not become independent enough to be offered discharge despite an intensive programme of care on the part of all those in the multi-disciplinary team who had contact with her.

Observation

It was important for the nurses not to lose heart and give up on Constance. They had to find purpose in the care they offered, and be able to see the effects it had upon her. This was achieved by regulating her activities, progress and potential, and correlating them against her known nursing diagnosis, objectives and nursing intervention. However, after 12 months of in-patient care, it became necessary to evaluate the whole of her presentation with particular reference to the approach and objectives used by the nursing team. At a weekly care review meeting the primary nurse responsible for Constance's care presented the following observational material.

Physiological

1 Relatively immobile, sitting in her chair most of the day and reluctant to take any form of physical exercise.

2 Poor attention to personal hygiene. Will only wash or bathe under supervision.

3 Poor dietary intake. Anaemia marginally controlled by monitoring her daily nutrition, with added iron tablets, but eats little unless encouraged.

4 Fluid intake restricted to an average of 500ml per day (tea).

5 Has a constant problem with constipation which causes her abdominal pain and discomfort.

6 Incontinent of urine if nursing intervention is removed.

7 Has become increasingly unsafe on her feet if left to walk unattended. This unsteady gait appears to be a result of loss of strength rather than problems of balance. Muscle wastage noted in both thighs and arms.

8 Gradual but persistent weight loss of 14 kilos noted over the last 12 months (on

admission weighed 61 kilos now weighs 47 kilos).

9   Has been prone to respiratory infections during the past 12 months (on four occasions). Treated successfully with various antibiotics.

Psychological

1   Appears unaware of her surroundings and relatively ambivalent to what goes on around her.

2   Does not seem to know where she is, who other people are, frequently misidentifying them, nor has she any appreciation of time.

3   Cannot remember recent events. Has a memory span of no more than 15 seconds. Can remember events and experiences relevant to her from childhood up until her late 50s, but these are all of a subjective nature.

4   Tends to confabulate, or make things up without realising she is doing so when her memory lets her down. It is as if she realises there is a gap in her memory and places, what is for her, the most logical answer in its place.

Confabulation is an unconscious process found in many organic psychoses where failings in memory are filled by stories, facts or data which seem appropriate. In this way the individual compensates for his/her memory defect

5   Appears to feel sad and looks emotionally flattened. Does not experience a full range of emotional responses.

6   Tends to be impulsive at times, often acting without recourse to the rather dangerous consequences of her behaviour.

7   Has a limited concentration span of no more than several minutes.

8   Is restless and agitated at times, especially in the company of other patients.

9   Is suspicious of others, often accusing people of stealing from her. The items she feels are stolen are not in her current possession but seem to have been part of her possessions at one time or other.

10 Feels anxious and has a low self esteem.
11 There appears to be some evidence of visual and auditory hallucinations especially when she has remained withdrawn for periods of time.

Sociological

1 Although her vocabulary remains quite intact, she speaks very little to others except to accuse them of various crimes against her. In response to conversational approaches, her response is usually monotoned or monosyllabic.
2 Is lonely and obviously misses her husband. She appears unaware of his death, often stating she has to go home to make his tea, or incorrectly identifying male members of staff as him.
3 Hoards apparently worthless pieces of paper in her clothing and items belonging to other people in her handbag. As a consequence of this, often gets into violent arguments with fellow patients.

Positive observations

1 She can walk quite well if supported and will use a walking frame.
2 Responds to encouragement to eat and drink well.
3 Can still read, and enjoys listening to the radio.
4 Enjoys looking at, and talking about, photographs which depict scenes she might have been familiar with when she was younger (reminiscence therapy).
5 Enjoys constant attention from nursing personnel when she is not put to the test about her memory, or any other gap in her need satisfaction. She likes being made to feel important.
6 Seems happiest when on ward outings and becomes quite 'chatty' on the bus.
7 Has no financial problems. All her belongings from the flat are with her on the ward,

and her quite considerable financial assets are held in trust by the Court of Protection.

Explanatory note: under Mental Health Legislation, people admitted to hospital who are considered by their consultant to have either a temporary or permanent inability to handle their affairs to their own benefit may have their affairs looked after by a central body known as the Court of Protection. This legal body usually appoints a suitable trustee to manage financial obligations until such time as the individual is well enough to do so for himself once again. The trustee is often a close relative, but in Constance's case, as she has no known relatives, it might well be the family solicitor. The trustee must ensure that the individual has all the financial support he or she needs while unwell, in line with their actual resources, and must provide the Court of Protection with regular accounts. The sums involved are immaterial, ranging from small 'nest eggs' to massive capital expenditures in the case of big business. The object of the Court is always the same, to protect the individual's estate and social balance so that he does not become financially disadvantaged because of mental illness.

NURSING CARE

Assessment

The main priorities of Constance's care at this time were seen as:

1 Promoting exercise
2 Helping her orientation and memory difficulties
3 Improving her social contact

The positive aspects in her profile must be considered so that any attempts to increase her ability will be centred around those items which give her the most satisfying reinforcement. It was significant that despite quite a concerted effort on the part of the nursing team to maintain Constance's level of performance, she had become weaker, and more withdrawn during her stay in hospital, and her level of general mental functioning had deteriorated in line with this. The nurses must recognise that Constance would not improve

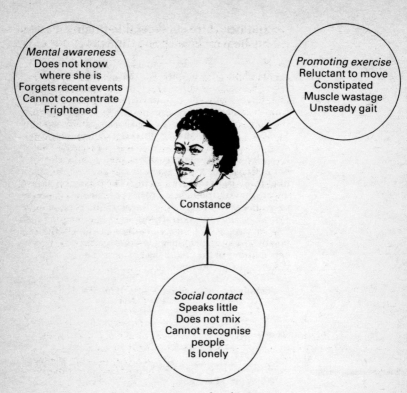

Mental awareness
Does not know
where she is
Forgets recent events
Cannot concentrate
Frightened

Promoting exercise
Reluctant to move
Constipated
Muscle wastage
Unsteady gait

Constance

Social contact
Speaks little
Does not mix
Cannot recognise
people
Is lonely

Priority assessment data for Constance

markedly. Thus their main objective for care is to try and slow this gradual deterioration down to a more acceptable level while maintaining a quality of life for her that gives as much pleasure and satisfaction as possible.

The selection of priorities for care reflected the view that many of Constance's problems revolved around her inability to orientate herself to her surroundings. She would not move about too much for fear of becoming even more lost, probably becoming confused and disoriented, and not mixing with others because she saw her failure to identify them as threatening. If these areas could be improved upon even a little, it would reduce some of her

anxiety and create a more meaningful environment in which to spend the remainder of her
life.

Explanatory note: many problems identified by nurses
are of secondary consequence. It is important that the
nurse try to identify the priority problems and needs;
often successful intervention with them can mean that
secondary ones are also resolved. Of course this is not
always the case but it would be impossible for nursing
staff to offer almost continuous nursing facilities and
resources to one patient in an attempt to meet all her
needs when there may be as many as 20 to 25 other
patients requiring a similar input into their daily care on
the same ward. The team have to rationalise what they
can offer so that each patient receives attention to their
priorities, either gradually increasing their own
capabilities or achieving a dignified decline with all the
respect and lack of disappointment that they deserve.

Possible consequences of Constance's care

Primary

Secondary problems
Constipation
Muscle wastage
Loss of physical strength
Increase in *mobility* and
exercise may improve ──────► Lack of interest in food/drink
Lack of orientation
Lack of interest in surroundings
Liability to chest infections
Incontinence of urine

Feeling sad and disinterested
Confabulation
Limited concentration
Increased performance in   Possible hallucinatory problems
orientation and *memory* may   Loneliness
improve ──────────────────► Feelings of anxiety
Lack of self esteem
Incontinence of urine

Loneliness/sadness
Lack of self esteem
Feelings of anxiety
Increase in *social contact*   Limited concentration
may improve ──────────────► Suspicion of others
Poor use of speech capabilities
Reduced sense of belonging

The therapy offered by the occupational team
has to be of a nature that can be reinforced by
nursing staff while Constance is on the ward.

It was thought advisable that she should attend regular sessions in the wards OT room rather than that in the central unit, as such a change in her environment might further increase her disorientation.

The psychologist had established through psychometric testing that Constance's cognitive abilities were greater than those she actually exhibited in her daily activities, so it was fair to assume that some slight improvement could be achieved if the right nursing intervention was selected. Review of medication by the medical staff did not find any necessity for change, though an increase in her existing anti-depressants was considered should her mood fail to lift with the alteration of her care.

Cognitive abilities are thinking processes including memory, concentration, analysis, decision making

NURSING CARE

Objectives

The team knew that it would be wrong to assume that Constance was unable to comprehend what was happening to her, even if she could not remember it. They therefore decided to discuss with her their intentions at regularly designated intervals, always being sure to employ simple unambiguous phrases that could be easily understood in their own right. The response they received from her was quite unexpected as she paid great attention to what was being said, even asking questions of them. True she did not seem to remember the conversations when next they spoke but each time she behaved in exactly the same fashion.

They initially set her objectives in each of the main areas as maintaining exactly the performance she presented at that time. In this way, they hoped to be able to achieve some form of immediate success upon which both she and they could build.

Intervention

The care being offered to Constance can be separated into two main areas, those of a personal approach and those of formal therapy. The method adopted on a personal level acts as the medium through which the formal therapy will be offered, so it is necessary to outline this in detail to ensure that all members of the primary team used the same techniques.

Personal approach

The following were principles of care adopted by all team members on the ward who came into contact with Constance.

1   When approaching Constance, always do so from the front, do not surprise her, or speak from a distance.

2   Place yourself at eye level with her at approximately arm's length, and place your hand on her shoulder if she will allow it. This should indicate to her that you intend to speak with her and her alone thus reducing any possible confusion.

3   Exaggerate facial mannerisms and make your actions simple but obvious.

4   All non-verbal behaviour should be exactly as you intend it. Do not use behaviour that can be misunderstood or misconstrued.

5   State simply and precisely what you wish to communicate without ambiguous or facetious comments. Use short words and do not be afraid to repeat yourself. If you detect from her countenance that she does not understand, use a different set of words.

6   Speak slowly and softly. Shouting is both threatening and more difficult to understand – she is not hard of hearing. Auditory sensory deprivation may well be

compounded if you increase the pitch of your voice by shouting. The ears of the elderly are more able to perceive lower pitched tones.

7 Always do what you say you are going to do. If you are unable to do so, explain why. Do not assume she will not remember as that is an insult to her integrity and intelligence.

8 Give her plenty of time to reply; do not interrupt her when she is speaking and listen carefully to what she says without being afraid to ask her to repeat herself.

9 Give her the opportunity to say and do things in her own way, and in her own time.

10 Observe the approaches and techniques used by other nurses. If they are successful in gaining positive responses from Constance, try and adopt the approach into existing methodology. If unsuccessful, discuss the reasons why.

11 Never assume that Constance is unable to do something – always give her the benefit, albeit under supervision or guidance, of competency.

Formal therapy
Several care activities and programmes existed on the ward and these were incorporated into Constance's specific care.

1 Her attention should be drawn to the pictures placed on walls and doors, etc. representing geographical areas around the ward. The use of pictures as signposts on wards for the elderly mentally ill is far more effective for helping patients orientate themselves. The visual impact is instant and easily understood, whereas with words, the reader has to go through an involved cognitive process which may confuse them, or they simply may not recog-

nise the words as significant.

2 Constance should be encouraged to attend both music appreciation and reminiscence therapy groups with a view to both occupying her time enjoyably and possibly reducing her suspicion of others.

3 An orientation card, stating the day's date, place, ward and any other relevant data should be placed in her handbag each morning. Night staff should ensure that a new card is made up for her each day. Should Constance seek any information that is contained on the card, nursing staff should refer her to the card rather than give her the answer.

4 A programme of personal contact ensures that Constance is either greeted or acknowledged at least once every 15 minutes during the day. Contact which does not require her to do anything, or where nothing is expected of her, endorses the sensation that she is among friends.

5 Discuss the contents of the local newspaper with her in the early evening. Particular reference should be made to local events, areas and well known places.

6 Provide Constance with any reading material she might like, and ascertain that she sits in a well lit chair to read. Ask her what she is reading. She particularly likes women's magazines.

7 Encourage a programme of both passive and active physiotherapy to be coordinated by the physiotherapist. Games or pursuits that involve moving of any nature should be encouraged. Constance must walk a prescribed distance, supervised and with a walking frame, at least once an hour. Incorporate this activity into other elements of her care programme where possible to avoid the risk of her carrying out seemingly meaningless physical exertions.

8 Ensure that she is kept warm when sitting inactively.

9 Weight chart, continence chart, conversational book (outlining the content of her conversations, likes, dislikes and responses, to be used as the basis for continuity in nurse interactions), a list of her dietary likes and dislikes, fluid intake chart and respirations must be maintained.

NURSING CARE

Evaluation

Every fortnight Constance's care plan was reviewed. At first there was a definite increase in her self help capabilities and especially her urinary incontinence which virtually ceased. The increase in personal contact appeared to have the most marked effect; because the quality of response she gave improved, the nursing intervention also reciprocated. It was possible to actually produce a series of 'increasing' objectives rather than decreasing ones, although eventually Constance reached a ceiling in her performance which she was never able to go above again. Gradually the team had to devise ways of maintaining her performance while reducing the amount of supervision they offered, allowing her the highest degree of dignity and self esteem possible. The greatest improvement area, which persisted for most of the time, was the lifting of her mood. She became much more tolerant and seemed an altogether happier person.

Other areas requiring regular evaluation to ensure the optimum effect of nursing intervention were her individual coping mechanisms, her level of awareness, her happiness and emotional responses and the appreciation of the quality of her life. It was hoped that the remainder of her stay in hospital, until her eventual death, would have meaning and a sense of purpose, with a personal commitment from Constance herself.

TEST YOURSELF

1 Outline the differences that exist between the normal ageing process and that considered to be abnormal.

2 Consider three priorities of elderly mentally ill people not listed in the chapter as such, and show how intervention in those areas might have a therapeutic effect on other secondary problems.

3 Describe a personalised approach programme for an elderly mentally ill individual and consider why it should be so important that such a programme exists.

4 What do you consider to be the most difficult problem facing nursing caring for the elderly mentally ill?

FURTHER READING

RIMMER, L. 1982. *Reality Orientation: Principles and Practice.* Winslow Press, Winslow, Bucks.
SUGDEN, J. & SAXBY, P. J. 1985. The confused elderly patient. *Nursing,* 2nd series, **35**: 1022–5.
WARD, M. F. 1985. The nursing process for the elderly mentally ill. Chapter 10 in *The Nursing Process in Psychiatry*: 181–90. Edinburgh: Churchill Livingstone.
ZACHOW, K. M. 1984. Helen, can you hear me? *Journal of Gerontological Nursing,* **10**, 8: 18–22.

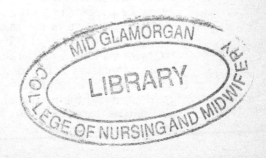

The Stages of Illness

Stage One

It could be argued that there are three separate stages to a psychiatric problem. The first is the construction, usually over a long period of time, of the problem itself. The individual will develop for himself various behaviour patterns that at first keep him out of trouble, probably by helping him avoid the problem. Gradually as the avoidance becomes more difficult to carry out, the behaviour becomes more involved and time consuming, resulting in other areas of his life being affected. Eventually others will begin to notice that he is in some kind of difficulty and hopefully lend a helping hand. Unfortunately a great many individuals find that their avoidance behaviour has left them with few real friends so the onus for help often lies with relatives. In this way the difficulties of psychiatric behaviour become a familiarised problem which leads to the whole family being affected in one way or another. Ultimately it is often the case that professional help is sought for the individual's problem by a relative rather than the individual himself. By the time this has happened, the behaviour adopted by the individual has become internalised. In other words, the behaviour has become a ritual or pattern naturally adopted and the individual can think of no alternative despite the fact that he is often distressed because of it.

Familiarised problem is a problem for each member of an individual's family, but affecting them all in different ways. Sometimes family members get so used to the presence of the problem, they are unaware of its effect on them

Stage Two

The second stage then begins with a consultation with one of the health professionals. It might be a social worker, district nurse or community psychiatric nurse, but it is most likely to be the family doctor. He will usually be confronted with the decision as to whether to treat the individual himself or refer him to a specialist. In a great many cases, the general practitioner will try to handle the situation himself but because he is unable to provide the necessary help, time or skills to confront the actual problem itself, he will have to treat the individual systematically. This involves either medication or minimal counselling for the effects of the problem which can range from mild depression and anxiety to panic attacks and a whole host of physiological symptoms such as skin rashes, shortness of breath, insomnia and impotence. As it is unable to get at the heart of the matter, this form of therapy has to be regarded as second best. However, at least the individual gains relief, no matter how superficial. Of course, that relief may not be enough for some individuals. Further changes in therapy may be available, especially if the general practitioner has a community psychiatric nurse attached to his clinic. The nurse may be in a position to visit the individual in his own home and give more insightful support by helping to isolate the true problem and then supplying guidance and teaching so that alternative methods of behaviour are sought and adopted.

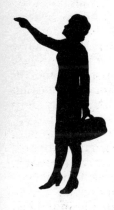

For a small minority of individuals, even this form of help is not enough and as we have seen in the preceding chapters, some period of hospitalisation then becomes the viable alternative. For some it will only be a short stay during which time they are able to consider their approaches to tackling their life problems in an objective and safe environment, culminating in a serious re-appraisal of themselves, and a return to the community with new hope and optimism. Others will spend longer in hospital, a few for months, even years. The treatment they receive may be long and involved, sorting out deep seated problems resulting from difficult childhoods, faulty learning of behaviour, poor personal relationships and personal insecurity. As a rule of thumb, it is fair to say that the longer it takes for psychiatric behaviour to develop to an intolerable level for the individual, the longer it will take to rehabilitate him to the point where he is able to lead an acceptable life style once again. Conversely, the shorter the onset of the condition, the quicker the recovery. As a consequence of this, people who have spent longer in psychiatric hospitals need far more support and rehabilitation, which in itself may take many years. Much of that rehabilitation work will be carried out in the hospital itself, and later in the community. The second stage has run its course when the problem has been successfully isolated and tackled. In truth, for many of the continuing care patients in psychiatric hospitals today, any real chance of a return to society will depend on the nature of the community resources available to them. It must be said that despite the tremendous advances made over the last 10 years in community services for ex-psychiatric patients, the general level of support remains patchy, depending on the individual health districts.

Stage Three
The third stage is, therefore, the successful rehabilitation process of any individual no matter how long his psychiatric behaviour has persisted, and the eventual resettling of him back into the community by the community team. At this point any number of alternatives are open to the individual. Depending on his

degree of recovery and his level of independence, he may be in a position to break contact with the community team altogether. However, in most cases this is neither likely or desirable. The reasons for this are simple. When an individual has been in hospital to regain his problem tackling ability, several problems will present on his discharge. These may range from a loss of real contact with the outside world, lack of understanding about what is going on around him or more obviously a lack in personal confidence derived from using new and often untried behaviour. Even if he has had the opportunity to put his new skills into practice before leaving hospital, which is usually the case, they will hardly have been tested in real situations that push him to the limit. Such situations are only likely to occur when he is on his own once again. It is, therefore, important that complete

Possible members of the community team

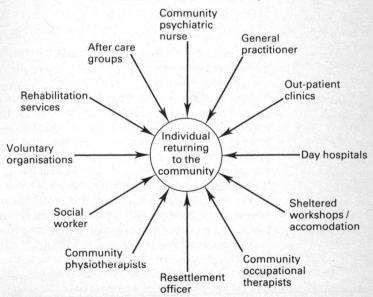

links with the support of the community team are not severed until he has regained his confidence. This can only be achieved by testing himself.

Possible consequences of discharge from hospital

Discharge from hospital
↓
Stigma
Lack of personal confidence
Poor self esteem
Poor social skills
Lack of personal assertiveness
Feelings of isolation/loneliness
Feelings of rejection
Unfamiliar surroundings
Changes within the community structure
Lack of occupation/recreation
Diminished motivation
Lack of finance
Inability to establish life routine
Possible return of psychiatric behaviour
↓
Re-admission to hospital

Role of the Community Team in the Third Stage

The various members of the community team have their own special roles to play in ensuring that the individual achieves a successful return to the community. If the rehabilitation process has been correctly organised, the individual will already have been in contact with team members before his discharge from hospital. Social workers, community psychiatric nurses, care groups and voluntary organisations may well have participated in the patient's activities organised while under inpatient supervision. These might include living for a period in a hostel ward where the individual retains patient status, but is responsible for the day to day running of the hostel and may even become employed while sleeping at the hostel. On a more superficial level, it might include shopping trips, outings to locate accommodation or simple re-orientation. The specific roles of each member of the team are too involved to discuss here, but the actual involvement of the community psychiatric nurse requires special attention.

The Community Psychiatric Nurse

If one accepts that the role of the community team in the successful rehabilitation of an individual from a psychiatric hospital requires them to create a situation in which the individual regains self direction and personal independence whilst retaining a sense of well being, how then can the nurse actively participate in this process? To answer this question fully, one must consider the two possible levels of achievement available to the individual that might be regarded as recovery. On the one hand, with full recovery the individual can anticipate a resumption of his life style without the burden of psychiatric problems. With limited recovery in which the individual has to learn to live with his problems as best he can, those psychiatric difficulties may persist and limit his ability to lead a fully independent life. He may find it more difficult to gain personal satisfaction. The community psychiatric nurse, therefore, has two separate roles to play in accordance with the degree of recovery.

Full Recovery

Here the nurse may visit the individual before discharge from hospital, introducing herself and explaining her support role for him when he leaves hospital. She will already be familiar with his care plan, and along with him she will identify how she is able to help him when this care plan ceases to be effective, i.e. on dis-

Two possible recovery courses available to the individual
on discharge from hospital

Recognition of problems	Identification of better problem tackling skills	Use of new skills	Improved life style	Mental health	Full recovery
Recognition of problems	Identification of better problem tackling skills	Limited ability to use new skills	Adapting life style accordingly	Learning to live with problems	Limited recovery

charge. She will construct a community care plan with him that will come into effect as soon as he leaves hospital. It might include times of her visits, the degree of support she will offer, the nature of her visits, e.g. for the giving of injections, simple counselling and monitoring of his performance. She will identify the involvement of relations and friends and her commitment to his continued improvement. She will show him how he can contact her, and when and why he would do so thus making herself available to him if he should need her. She will already be aware of the types of therapy that have brought about his recovery, the evaluations of his care objectives that have plotted his progress, and his new objectives will be set as a contract between herself and the individual. Finally she will describe how she will gradually reduce her input, as circumstances warrant, until he no longer requires her for either support, guidance, confidence boosting or medication. She will, however, indicate that this withdrawal of support is flexible and may be increased if the necessity arises.

Limited Recovery
The initial contact will be similar to that of the full recovery inidividual, although it may vary in intensity. The community psychiatric

nurse may spend more time with the limited recovery individual prior to discharge to establish a closer relationship, and give a clear picture of what special support and help is required of her.

The difference will become apparent once the individual has been discharged. It may well be that she will need to keep him as a member of her care group for an extremely long period of time, even indefinitely, and her in-put has to be geared towards his changing needs while living in the community. As the individual learns to adapt his life style to the ever present accompaniment of his problem, she too must monitor the effects of such an existence on his ability to regain independence and happiness. If he begins to lose his sense of achievement and purpose, becomes lonely, isolated and depressed, a return of psychiatric behaviour may be heralded in an attempt to avoid the anxiety experienced. Re-hospitalisation is not necessarily a sign of failure, but it may be seen to be so by the individual and it may take a far longer period of time to get him back into the community once again. The nurse's visits to him may have to be more frequent and longer time spent with him than with an individual who is hoping to achieve unqualified recovery.

It may be a necessary part of her job to administer regular injections, usually an average of about once a fortnight, of depot medications. These are long acting tranquillisers which help to level the individual's mood and remove psychiatric symptoms, i.e. hallucinations, and delusional systems, etc. In truth, the nurse's support and guidance plus the use of such medication may be the only reason that the individual is able to retain his place within the community.

The Changing Face of Community Care

The conclusion of this short chapter must briefly consider the way that community teams are beginning to have more significance within the care of individuals experiencing psychiatric problems. Since the beginning of the twentieth century, it has been an accepted principle that if beds are available in psychiatric hospitals, then suitable individuals will be found to occupy them. This rather cynical view is based on the fact that no viable alternative to hospitalisation was really available up until a few years ago when the popular belief of the day was challenged by an enlightened group of professionals who argued that care in the community, without actually admitting the individual at all was a more desirable method of care. They called this approach *crisis intervention* – in other words acting to solve the problem in the situation in which it occurred rather than compounding it by removing the individual to a hospital, which was in effect a false environment.

The growth of this approach coupled with the necessity to rehabilitate people who had been in psychiatric hospitals for far too long, the development of depot medication and other effective methods of therapies, an increase in the awareness of the need not to separate the individual from his own society and the realisation that hospital life could, in effect, create its own group of psychiatric behaviour problems (*institutionalisation*) brought about the emergence of an energetic community policy. Many health authorities in the UK are now following procedures that will eventually revolutionise the face of psychiatric care. Gradually fewer people are being admitted to psychiatric hospitals, and more are being discharged. Facilities traditionally available within a hospital setting, i.e. occupational therapy, physiotherapy and psychotherapy, are being re-organised and placed on a community footing so that they are directly available to those outside of hospital.

Only time will tell if this policy can reap the benefits for the individuals concerned that it promises at present. One thing, however, is certain. We all begin life in the community and no matter whether we are admitted to a psychiatric hospital or not, that remains our rightful place in society. If you are admitted to hospital, it is often a long and painful path which leads back into the community. If a positive and resourceful community team can reduce the time spent by individuals in psychiatric hospitals, this can only be seen as a step in the right direction.

FURTHER READING

DIXON, S. L. 1979. *Working with People in Crisis – Theory and Practice.* St Louis: Mosby.
FRAZER, F. N. (Ed.) 1982. *Rehabilitation within the Community.* London: Faber and Faber Ltd.
GOLDBERG, D. & HUXLEY, P. 1980. *Mental Illness in the Community. The Pathway to Psychiatric Care.* London: Tavistock.

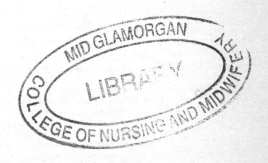

INDEX

Abnormal ageing 146
Abreaction 78
Actively suicidal 41
Anaemia 149–50
Anorexia nervosa 72, 73
Anxiety 24, 30
Anxiolytic 22, 45, 92
Aphonia 70
Art therapy 51
Assertiveness
    group 92
    training 50
Auditory hallucinations 64,
    103, 152
Auditory sensory
    deprivation 157

Biopsychosocial evaluation
    39, 70

Circumlocution 76
Clinical psychologist 2
Close contact care 41
Community psychiatric
    nurse 2
Compulsions 90
Confabulation 151
Conversational skills 138–
    40
Conversion 73
Court of Protection 153
Crisis intervention team 38
Cyclothymic personality
    120

Defence mechanisms 73
Delirium tremens 62
Delusion 64
Denial 76
Depot medication 99, 132
Depression 29, 38, 46, 47
Disorientation 64
Dissociation 73
Diurnal mood swing 46
Diversional therapy 51

Emotional seduction 76
Empathy 43
Extra-pyramidal tract 118,
    132

Facial mannerisms 157
Family guilt 131, 139
    therapy 112–13

General mental function
    153
Guilt 89, 131

Hierarchy of problems 31
Hostel ward 139
Hostility 76
Hysteria 72

Industrial therapy 142
Informal admission 7
Initial insomnia 46
Institutionalisation 141
Intellectualisation 76

La belle indifference 71

Malingering 73
Mania 99
Manic depressive illness
    125
Memory loss 151
Mental Health Act 7, 45,
    99, 101, 102
Modelling techniques 60
Mood, flattening 39
Munchausen syndrome 72,
    73
Music therapy 51, 159

Non-verbal behaviour 157
Nurses' uniform 15

Objective sequence 141
Observation section 45
Obsessions 90
Occupational therapy 31,
    95
    therapist 2, 142
Orientation card 159
Overt behaviour 15, 28

Paranoia 64
Passive physiotherapy 159
Patient/nurse relationship
    31, 41, 127
Patient progress 10
Personal assertiveness 136
    choice 111
Personality 10, 12, 13, 16
    disorder 59
Picture signposts 158
Positive features 45
Pre-morbid personality 70

Primary nursing team 29,
    31
Problem solving 138–41
Psychiatric first aid 29
Psychodrama 51, 60
Psychometric testing 156
Psychomotor retardation 39
Psychopath 59
Psychosis 98
Psychosomatic conditions
    73
Psychotherapy 75, 92
Psychotic depression 99

Rapport 13
Reality orientation 99, 111
Recreational therapies 51
Rehabilitation 130
    staff 2
Relaxation therapy 31, 50
REM sleep 46
Reminiscence therapy 152,
    159
Resettlement officer 2
Residual psychosis 143
Restraint 14
Rituals 85, 89, 131, 145
Role play 51

Schizophrenia 99, 106
Self awareness group 92
Self image 95
Senescence 146
Senile dementia 146
Sleep reversal 149
Social
    skills 51, 128
    worker 2
Speech 38
Splitting 73
Stigma 131
Suicidal ruminations 94
Superficiality 76

Thought stopping
    techniques 91

Verbal communication 134
Visual hallucinations 64,
    152
Volition 136

Warden controlled flat 148
Ward meetings 91
Withdrawal 76